Lecture Notes in Computer Science 11037

Commenced Publication in 1973
Founding and Former Series Editors:
Gerhard Goos, Juris Hartmanis, and Jan van Leeuwen

More information about this series at http://www.springer.com/series/7412

Ali Gooya · Orcun Goksel
Ipek Oguz · Ninon Burgos (Eds.)

Simulation and Synthesis in Medical Imaging

Third International Workshop, SASHIMI 2018
Held in Conjunction with MICCAI 2018
Granada, Spain, September 16, 2018
Proceedings

Springer

Editors
Ali Gooya (iD)
University of Sheffield
Sheffield
UK

Orcun Goksel (iD)
ETH Zurich
Zurich
Switzerland

Ipek Oguz (iD)
Vanderbilt University
Nashville, TN
USA

Ninon Burgos (iD)
Pitié-Salpêtrière Hospital
Paris
France

ISSN 0302-9743   ISSN 1611-3349   (electronic)
Lecture Notes in Computer Science
ISBN 978-3-030-00535-1   ISBN 978-3-030-00536-8   (eBook)
https://doi.org/10.1007/978-3-030-00536-8

Library of Congress Control Number: 2018954070

LNCS Sublibrary: SL6 – Image Processing, Computer Vision, Pattern Recognition, and Graphics

This Springer imprint is published by the registered company Springer Nature Switzerland AG
The registered company address is: Gewerbestrasse 11, 6330 Cham, Switzerland

Preface

The Medical Image Computing and Computer Assisted Intervention (MICCAI) community needs data with known ground truth to develop, evaluate, and validate image analysis and reconstruction algorithms. Since synthetic data are ideally suited for this purpose, over the years, a full range of models underpinning image simulation and synthesis have been developed: (i) deep learning based models for data generation and synthesis; (ii) mechanistic models, which incorporate priors on the geometry and physics of image acquisition and formation processes; and (iii) complex spatio-temporal computational models of anatomical variability, organ physiology, or disease progression.

The goal of the Simulation and Synthesis in Medical Imaging (SASHIMI)[1] workshop is to gather all those interested in these problems in the same room, for the purpose of invigorating research and stimulating new ideas on how to best proceed and bring these two worlds together. The objectives were to (a) hear from invited speakers in the areas of machine learning and mechanistic models; (b) bring together experts of synthesis and simulation to raise the state of the art; and (c) identify challenges and opportunities for further research. We also wanted to identify how we can best evaluate synthetic data and if we could collect benchmark data that can help the development of future algorithms.

The third SASHIMI workshop was successfully held in conjunction with the 21st International Conference on Medical Image Computing and Computer-Assisted Intervention (MICCAI 2018) as a satellite event in Granada, Spain, on September 16, 2018. Submissions were solicited via a call for papers that was circulated by the MICCAI organizers, through known mailing lists but also by directly emailing several colleagues and experts in the area. Each submission underwent a double-blind review by at least two members of the Program Committee consisting of researchers who actively contribute in the area. At the conclusion of the review process, 14 papers were accepted. Overall, the contributions span the following broad categories in alignment with the initial call for papers: deep learning methods for MRI/MRS/CT image synthesis/generation, time-lapse generation, cell and tubular network generation, and several applications of image synthesis and simulation for data augmentation. The accepted papers were divided into two general topics of "Synthesis and Its Applications in Computational Medical Imaging" and "Simulation and Processing Approaches for Medical Imaging" and presented within one oral and one poster sessions, overall covering 6 and 8 papers, respectively.

Finally, we would like to thank everyone who contributed to this third workshop: members of the Organizing Committee for their assistance; the authors for their contributions; the members of the Program Committee for their review work, promotion

---

[1] http://www.sashimi.aramislab.fr.

of the workshop, and general support; the invited speaker, Prof. Olaf Ronneberger, for sharing his expertise and knowledge; and the MICCAI society for the general support.

August 2018   Ali Gooya
                                                                                  Orcun Goksel
                                                                                      Ipek Oguz
                                                                                  Ninon Burgos

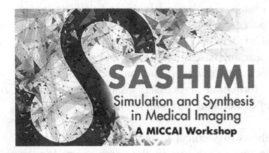

Organization

Organizing Committee

Ali Gooya   University of Sheffield, UK
Orcun Goksel   ETH Zurich, Switzerland
Ipek Oguz   Vanderbilt University, USA
Ninon Burgos   Inria Paris, France

Steering Committee

Sotirios A. Tsaftaris   University of Edinburgh, UK
Alejandro F. Frangi   University of Leeds, UK
Jerry L. Prince   Johns Hopkins University, USA

Program Committee

Ninon Burgos   Inria Paris, France
Aaron Carass   John Hopkins University, USA
Orcun Goksel   ETH Zurich, Switzerland
Ali Gooya   University of Sheffield, UK
Daniel Herzka   John Hopkins University, USA
Jack Noble   Vanderbilt University, USA
Ipek Oguz   Vanderbilt University, USA
Dzung L. Pham   National Institutes of Health, USA
Adityo Prakosa   John Hopkins University, USA
Snehashis Roy   National Institutes of Health, USA
Devrim Unay   Izmir University of Economics, Turkey
François Varray   CREATIS, France

Contents

Medical Image Synthesis for Data Augmentation and Anonymization Using Generative Adversarial Networks

Hoo-Chang Shin[1]([✉]), Neil A. Tenenholtz[2], Jameson K. Rogers[2],
Christopher G. Schwarz[3], Matthew L. Senjem[3], Jeffrey L. Gunter[3],
Katherine P. Andriole[2], and Mark Michalski[2]

[1] NVIDIA Corporation, Santa Clara, USA
hshin@nvidia.com
[2] MGH & BWH Center for Clinical Data Science, Boston, MA, USA
{ntenenholtz,jrogers24}@partners.org
[3] Mayo Clinic, Rochester, MN, USA
gunter.jeffrey@mayo.edu

Abstract. Data diversity is critical to success when training deep learning models. Medical imaging data sets are often imbalanced as pathologic findings are generally rare, which introduces significant challenges when training deep learning models. In this work, we propose a method to generate synthetic abnormal MRI images with brain tumors by training a generative adversarial network using two publicly available data sets of brain MRI. We demonstrate two unique benefits that the synthetic images provide. First, we illustrate improved performance on tumor segmentation by leveraging the synthetic images as a form of data augmentation. Second, we demonstrate the value of generative models as an anonymization tool, achieving comparable tumor segmentation results when trained on the synthetic data versus when trained on real subject data. Together, these results offer a potential solution to two of the largest challenges facing machine learning in medical imaging, namely the small incidence of pathological findings, and the restrictions around sharing of patient data.

Keywords: Generative models · GAN · Image synthesis
Deep learning · Brain tumor · Magnetic resonance imaging · MRI
Segmentation

1 Introduction

It is widely known that sufficient data volume is necessary for training a successful machine learning algorithm [6] for medical image analysis. Data with high class imbalance or of insufficient variability [18] leads to poor classification performance. This often proves to be problematic in the field of medical imaging where abnormal findings are by definition uncommon. Moreover, in the case of

© Springer Nature Switzerland AG 2018
A. Gooya et al. (Eds.): SASHIMI 2018, LNCS 11037, pp. 1–11, 2018.
https://doi.org/10.1007/978-3-030-00536-8_1

image segmentation tasks, the time required to manually annotate volumetric data only exacerbates this disparity; manually segmenting an abnormality in three dimensions can require upwards of fifteen minutes per study making it impractical in a busy radiology practice. The result is a paucity of annotated data and considerable challenges when attempting to train an accurate algorithm. While traditional data augmentation techniques (e.g., crops, translation, rotation) can mitigate some of these issues, they fundamentally produce highly correlated image training data.

In this paper we demonstrate one potential solution to this problem by generating synthetic images using a generative adversarial network (GAN) [9], which provides an additional form of data augmentation and also serves as a effective method of data anonymization. Multi-parametric magnetic resonance images (MRIs) of abnormal brains (with tumor) are generated from segmentation masks of brain anatomy and tumor. This offers an automatable, low-cost source of diverse data that can be used to supplement the training set. For example, we can alter the tumor's size, change its location, or place a tumor in an otherwise healthy brain, to systematically have the image and the corresponding annotation. Furthermore, GAN trained on a hospital data to generate synthetic images can be used to share the data outside of the institution, to be used as an anonymization tool.

Medical image simulation and synthesis have been studied for a while and are increasingly getting traction in medical imaging community [7]. It is partly due to the exponential growth in data availability, and partly due to the availability of better machine learning models and supporting systems. Twelve recent research on medical image synthesis and simulation were presented in the special issue of Simulation and Synthesis in Medical Imaging [7].

This work falls into the synthesis category, and most related works are those of Chartsias et al. [3] and Costa et al. [4]. We use the publicly available data set (ADNI and BRATS) to demonstrate multi-parametric MRI image synthesis and Chartsias et al. [3] use BRATS and ISLES (Ischemic Stroke Lesion Segmentation (ISLES) 2015 challenge) data set. Nonetheless, evaluation criteria for synthetic images were demonstrated on MSE, SSIM, and PSNR, but not directly on diagnostic quality. Costa et al. [4] used GAN to generate synthetic retinal images with labels, but the ability to represent more diverse pathological pattern was limited compared to this work. Also, both previous works were demonstrated on 2D images or slices/views of 3D images, whereas in this work we directly process 3D input/output. The input/output dimension is 4D when it is multi-parametric (T1/T2/T1c/Flair). We believe processing data as 3D/4D in nature better reflects the reality of data and their associated problems.

Reflecting the general trend of the machine learning community, the use of GANs in medical imaging has increased dramatically in the last year. GANs have been used to generate a motion model from a single preoperative MRI [10], upsample a low-resolution fundus image [13], create a synthetic head CT from a brain MRI [16], and synthesizing T2-weight MRI from T1-weighted ones (and vice-versa) [5]. Segmentation using GANs was demonstrated in [21,22].

Finally, Frid-Adar *et al.* leveraged a GAN for data augmentation, in the context of liver lesion classification [8]. To the best of our knowledge, there is no existing literature on the generation of synthetic medical images as form of anonymization and data augmentation for tumor segmentation tasks.

2 Data

2.1 Dataset

We use two publicly available data set of brain MRI:

Alzheimer's Disease Neuroimaging Initiative (ADNI) Data Set
The ADNI was launched in 2003 as a public-private partnership, led by principal investigator Michael W. Weiner, MD. The primary goal of ADNI has been to test whether serial magnetic resonance imaging (MRI), positron emission tomography (PET), other biological markers, and clinical and neuropsychological assessment can be combined to measure the progression of mild cognitive impairment (MCI) and early Alzheimer's disease (AD). For up-to-date information on the ADNI study, see www.adni-info.org. We follow the approach of [17] that is shown to be effective for segmenting the brain atlas of ADNI data. The atlas of white matter, gray matter, and cerebrospinal fluid (CSF) in the ADNI T1-weighted images are generated using the SPM12 [1] segmentation and the ANTs SyN [19] non-linear registration algorithms. In total, there are 3,416 pairs of T1-weighted MRI and their corresponding segmented tissue class images.

Multimodal Brain Tumor Image Segmentation Benchmark (BRATS) Data Set
BRATS utilizes multi-institutional pre-operative MRIs and focuses on the segmentation of intrinsically heterogeneous (in appearance, shape, and histology) brain tumors, namely gliomas [14]. Each patient's MRI image set includes a variety of series including T1-weighted, T2-weighted, contrast-enhanced T1, and FLAIR, along with a ground-truth voxel-wise annotation of edema, enhancing tumor, and non-enhancing tumor. For more details about the BRATS data set, see braintumorsegmentation.org. While the BRATS challenge is held annually, we used the BRATS 2015 training data set which is publicly available.

2.2 Dataset Split and Pre-processing

As a pre-processing step, we perform skull-stripping [11] on the ADNI data set as skulls are not present in the BRATS data set. The BRATS 2015 training set provides 264 studies, of which we used the first 80% as a training set, and the remaining 20% as a test set to assess final algorithm performance. Hyperparameter optimization was performed within the training set and the test set was evaluated only once for each algorithm and settings assessed. Our GAN operates in 3D, and due to memory and compute constraints, training images were cropped axially to include the central 108 slices, discarding those above and below this central region, then resampled to $128 \times 128 \times 54$ for model training and inference. For a fair evaluation of the segmentation performance to the BRATS challenge we used the original images with a resolution of $256 \times 256 \times 108$ for evaluation and comparison. However, it is possible that very small tumor may get lost by the downsampling, thus affecting the final segmentation performance.

3 Methods

The image-to-image translation conditional GAN (`pix2pix`) model introduced in [12] is adopted to translate label-to-MRI (synthetic image generation) and MRI-to-label (image segmentation). For brain segmentation, the generator G is given a T1-weighted image of ADNI as input and is trained to produce a brain mask with white matter, grey matter and CSF. The discriminator D on the other hand, is trained to distinguish "real" labels versus synthetically generated "fake" labels. During the procedure (depicted in Fig. 1(a)) the generator G learns to segment brain labels from a T1-weighted MRI input. Since we did not have an appropriate off-the-shelf segmentation method available for brain anatomy in the BRATS data set, and the ADNI data set does not contain tumor information, we first train the `pix2pix` model to segment normal brain anatomy from the T1-weighted images of the ADNI data set. We then use this model to perform inference on the T1 series of the BRATS data set. The segmentation of neural anatomy, in combination with tumor segmentations provided by the BRATS data set, provide a complete segmentation of the brain with tumor. The synthetic image generation is trained by reversing the inputs to the generator and training the discriminator to perform the inverse task (i.e., "is this imaging data

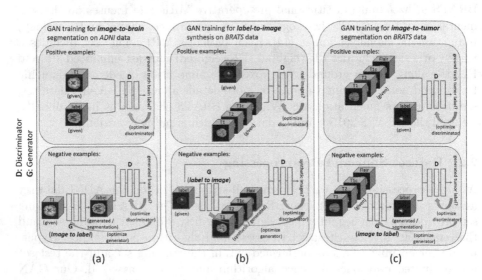

Fig. 1. Illustration of training GAN for (a) MRI-to-brain segmentation; (b) label-to-MRI synthesis; (c) MRI-to-tumor segmentation.

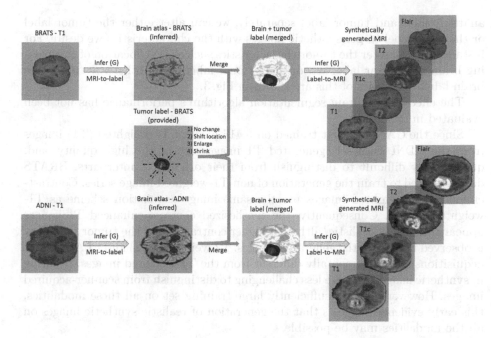

Fig. 2. Workflow of getting synthetic images with variation. On BRATS data set, MRI-to-label image translation GAN is applied to T1-weighted images to get brain atlas. It is then merged with the tumor label given in the BRATS data set, possibly with alterations (shift tumor location; enlarge; shrink). The merged labels (with possibly alterations) are then used as an input to label-to-MRI GAN, to generate synthetic multi-parametric MRI with brain tumor.

acquired from a scanner or synthetically generated?" as opposed to "is this segmentation the ground-truth annotation or synthetically generated?" – Fig. 1(b)). We generate synthetic abnormal brain MRI from the labels and introduce variability by adjusting those labels (e.g., changing tumor size, moving the tumor's location, or placing tumor on a otherwise tumor-free brain label). Then GAN segmentation module is used once again, to segment tumor from the BRATS data set (input: multi-parametric MRI; output: tumor label). We compare the segmentation performance *(1)* with and without additional synthetic data, *(2)* using only the synthetic data and fine-tuning the model on 10% of the real data; and compare their performance of GAN to a top-performing algorithm[1] [20] from the BRATS 2017 challenge.

3.1   Data Augmentation with Synthetic Images

The GAN trained to generate synthetic images from labels allows for the generation of arbitrary multi-series abnormal brain MRIs. Since we have the brain

---

[1] https://github.com/taigw/brats17.

anatomy label and tumor label separately, we can alter either the tumor label or the brain label to get synthetic images with the characteristics we desire. For instance, we can alter the tumor characteristics such as size, location of the existing brain and tumor label set, or place tumor label on an otherwise tumor-free brain label. Examples of this are shown in Fig. 3.

The effect of the brain segmentation algorithm's performance has not been evaluated in this study.

Since the GAN was first trained on 3,416 pairs of T1-weighted (T1) images from the ADNI data set, generated T1 images are of the high quality, and, qualitatively difficult to distinguish from their original counterparts. BRATS data was used to train the generation of non-T1-weighted image series. Contrast-enhanced T1-weighted images use the same image acquisition scheme as T1-weighted images. Consequently, the synthesized contrast-enhanced T1 images appear reasonably realistic, although higher contrast along the tumor boundary is observed in some of the generated images. T2-weighted (T2) and FLAIR image acquisitions are fundamentally different from the T1-weighted images, resulting in synthetic images that are less challenging to distinguish from scanner-acquired images. However, given a sufficiently large training set on all these modalities, this early evidence suggests that the generation of realistic synthetic images on all the modalities may be possible.

Other than increasing the image resolution and getting more data especially for the sequences other than T1-weighted images, there are still a few important avenues to explore to improve the overall image quality. For instance, more attention likely needs to be paid for the tumor boundaries so it does not look superimposed and discrete when synthetic tumor is placed. Also, performance of brain segmentation algorithm and its ability to generalize across different data sets needs to be examined to obtain higher quality synthetic images combining data sets from different patient population.

The augmentation using synthetic images can be used in addition to the usual data augmentation methods such as random cropping, rotation, translation, or elastic deformation [15]. Moreover, we have more control over the augmented images using the GAN-based synthetic image generation approach, that we have more input-option (i.e., label) to perturb the given image than the usual data augmentation techniques. The usual data augmentation methods rely mostly on random processes and operates on the whole image level than specific to a location, such as tumor. Additionally, since we generate image from the corresponding label, we get more images for training without needing to go through the labor-intensive manual annotation process. Figure 4 shows the process of training GAN with real and synthetic image and label pairs.

3.2   Generating Anonymized Synthetic Images with Variation

Protection of personal health information (PHI) is a critical aspect of working with patient data. Often times concern over dissemination of patient data restricts the data availability to the research community, hindering development of the field. While removing all DICOM metadata and skull-stripping will

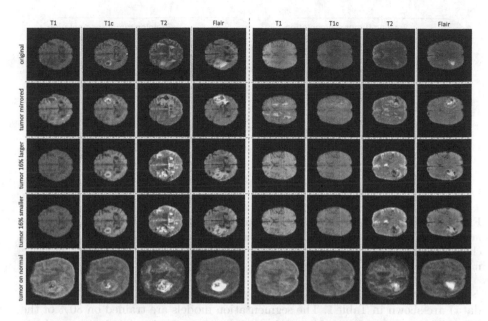

Fig. 3. Examples of generated images. The first row depicts the original ("real") images on which the synthetic tumors were based. Generated images without adjustment of the segmentation label are shown in the second row. Examples of generated images with various adjustments to the tumor segmentation label are shown in the third through fifth rows. The last row depicts examples of synthetic images where a tumor label is placed on a tumor-free brain label from the ADNI data set.

often eliminate nearly all identifiable information, demonstrably proving this to a hospital's data sharing committee is near impossible. Simply de-identifying the data is insufficient. Furthermore, models themselves are subject to caution when derived from sensitive patient data. It has been shown [2] that private data can be extracted from a trained model.

Development of a GAN that generates synthetic, but realistic, data may address these challenges. The first two rows of Fig. 3 illustrate how, even with the same segmentation mask, notable variations can be observed between the generated and original studies. This indicates that the GAN produces images that do not reflect the underlying patients as individuals, but rather draws individuals from the population in aggregate. It generates new data that cannot be attributed to a single patient but rather an instantiation of the training population conditioned upon the provided segmentation.

4   Experiments and Results

4.1   Data Augmentation Using Synthetic Data

Dice score evaluation of the whole tumor segmentation produced by the GAN-based model and the model of Wang *et al.* [20] (trained on real and synthetic

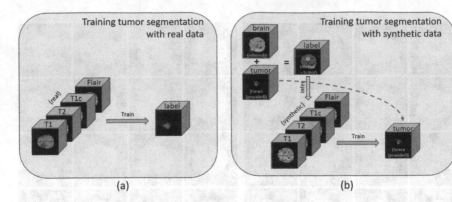

Fig. 4. Training GAN for tumor segmentation with (a) real; and (b) synthetic image-label pairs. Synthetic data generation can increase the training data set with desired characteristics (e.g., tumor size, location, etc.) without the need of labor-intensive manual annotation.

data) are shown in Table 1. The segmentation models are trained on 80% of the BRATS'15 training data only, and the training data supplemented with synthetic data. Dice scores are evaluated on the 20% held-out set from the BRATS'15 training data. All models are trained for 200 epochs on NVIDIA DGX systems.

A much improved performance with the addition of synthetic data is observed without usual data augmentation (crop, rotation, elastic deformation; GAN-based (no-aug)). However, a small increase in performance is observed when added with usual data augmentation (GAN-based (no-aug)), and it applies also to the model of Wang *et al.* [20] that incorporates usual data augmentation techniques.

Wang *et al.* model operates in full resolution (256×256) combining three 2D models for each axial/coronal/sagittal view, whereas our model and generator operates in half the resolution ($128 \times 128 \times 54$) due to GPU memory limit. We up-sampled the GAN-generated images twice the generated resolution for a fair comparison with BRATS challenge, however it is possible that very small tumor may get lost during the down-/up- sampling. A better performance may be observed using the GAN-based model with an availability of GPU with more memory. Also, we believe that the generated synthetic images having half the resolution, coupled with the lack of the image sequences for training other than T1-weighted ones possibly led to the relatively small increase in segmentation performance compared to using the usual data augmentation techniques. We carefully hypothesize that with more T2/Flair images being available, better image quality will be observed for these sequences and so better performance for more models and tumor types.

4.2   Training on Anonymized Synthetic Data

We also evaluated the performance of the GAN-based segmentation on synthetic data only, in amounts greater than or equal to the amount of real data but without including any of the original data. The dice score evaluations are shown in Table 1. Sub-optimal performance is achieved for both our GAN-based and the model of Wang *et al.* [20] when training on an amount of synthetic data equal to the original 80% training set. However, higher performance, comparable to training on real data, is achieved when training the two models using more than five times as much synthetic data (only), and fine-tuning using a 10% random selection of the "real" training data. In this case, the synthetic data provides a form of pre-training, allowing for much less "real" data to be used to achieve a comparable level of performance.

Table 1. Dice score evaluation (mean/standard deviation) of GAN-based segmentation algorithm and BRATS'17 top-performing algorithm [20], trained on "real" data only; real + synthetic data; and training on synthetic data only and fine-tuning the model on 10% of the real data. GAN-based models were trained both with (with aug) and without (no aug) including the usual data augmentation techniques (crop, rotation, translation, and elastic deformation) during training. All models were trained for 200 epochs to convergence.

Method	Real	Real + Synthetic	Synthetic only	Synthetic only, fine-tune on 10% real
GAN-based (no aug)	0.64/0.14	0.80/0.07	0.25/0.14	0.80/0.18
GAN-based (with aug)	0.81/0.13	0.82/0.08	0.44/0.16	0.81/0.09
Wang *et al.* [20]	0.85/0.15	0.86/0.09	0.66/0.13	0.84/0.15

5   Conclusion

In this paper, we propose a generative algorithm to produce synthetic abnormal brain tumor multi-parametric MRI images from their corresponding segmentation masks using an image-to-image translation GAN. High levels of variation can be introduced when generating such synthetic images by altering the input label map. This results in improvements in segmentation performance across multiple algorithms. Furthermore, these same algorithms can be trained on completely anonymized data sets allowing for sharing of training data. When combined with smaller, institution-specific data sets, modestly sized organizations are provided the opportunity to train successful deep learning models.

References

1. Ashburner, J., Friston, K.J.: Unified segmentation. Neuroimage **26**(3), 839–851 (2005)
2. Carlini, N., Liu, C., Kos, J., Erlingsson, Ú., Song, D.: The secret sharer: measuring unintended neural network memorization & extracting secrets. arXiv preprint arXiv:1802.08232 (2018)
3. Chartsias, A., Joyce, T., Giuffrida, M.V., Tsaftaris, S.A.: Multimodal MR synthesis via modality-invariant latent representation. IEEE Trans. Med. Imaging **37**(3), 803–814 (2018)
4. Costa, P.: End-to-end adversarial retinal image synthesis. IEEE Trans. Med. Imaging **37**(3), 781–791 (2018)
5. Dar, S.U.H., Yurt, M., Karacan, L., Erdem, A., Erdem, E., Çukur, T.: Image synthesis in multi-contrast MRI with conditional generative adversarial networks. arXiv preprint arXiv:1802.01221 (2018)
6. Domingos, P.: A few useful things to know about machine learning. Commun. ACM **55**(10), 78–87 (2012)
7. Frangi, A.F., Tsaftaris, S.A., Prince, J.L.: Simulation and synthesis in medical imaging. IEEE Trans. Med. Imaging **37**(3), 673–679 (2018)
8. Frid-Adar, M., Klang, E., Amitai, M., Goldberger, J., Greenspan, H.: Synthetic data augmentation using GAN for improved liver lesion classification. In: IEEE International Symposium on Biomedical Imaging (ISBI) (2018)
9. Goodfellow, I., et al.: Generative adversarial nets. In: Advances in Neural Information Processing Systems, pp. 2672–2680 (2014)
10. Hu, Y., et al.: Intraoperative organ motion models with an ensemble of conditional generative adversarial networks. In: Descoteaux, M., et al. (eds.) MICCAI 2017 Part II. LNCS, vol. 10434, pp. 368–376. Springer, Cham (2017). https://doi.org/10.1007/978-3-319-66185-8_42
11. Iglesias, J.E., Liu, C.-Y., Thompson, P.M., Tu, Z.: Robust brain extraction across datasets and comparison with publicly available methods. IEEE Trans. Med. Imaging **30**(9), 1617–1634 (2011)
12. Isola, P., Zhu, J.-Y., Zhou, T., Efros, A.A.: Image-to-image translation with conditional adversarial networks. In: The IEEE Conference on Computer Vision and Pattern Recognition (CVPR), July 2017
13. Mahapatra, D., Bozorgtabar, B., Hewavitharanage, S., Garnavi, R.: Image super resolution using generative adversarial networks and local saliency maps for retinal image analysis. In: Descoteaux, M., Maier-Hein, L., Franz, A., Jannin, P., Collins, D.L., Duchesne, S. (eds.) MICCAI 2017 Part III. LNCS, vol. 10435, pp. 382–390. Springer, Cham (2017). https://doi.org/10.1007/978-3-319-66179-7_44
14. Menze, B.H., et al.: The multimodal brain tumor image segmentation benchmark (BRATS). IEEE Trans. Med. Imaging **34**(10), 1993–2024 (2015)
15. Milletari, F., Navab, N., Ahmadi, S.-A.: V-net: fully convolutional neural networks for volumetric medical image segmentation. In: 2016 Fourth International Conference on 3D Vision (3DV), pp. 565–571. IEEE (2016)
16. Nie, D., et al.: Medical image synthesis with context-aware generative adversarial networks. In: Descoteaux, M., Maier-Hein, L., Franz, A., Jannin, P., Collins, D.L., Duchesne, S. (eds.) MICCAI 2017 Part III. LNCS, vol. 10435, pp. 417–425. Springer, Cham (2017). https://doi.org/10.1007/978-3-319-66179-7_48
17. Christopher, G.S., et al.: A large-scale comparison of cortical thickness and volume methods for measuring Alzheimer's disease severity. NeuroImage: Clin. **11**, 802–812 (2016)

18. Shin, H.-C., et al.: Deep convolutional neural networks for computer-aided detection: CNN architectures, dataset characteristics and transfer learning. IEEE Trans. Med. Imaging **35**(5), 1285–1298 (2016)
19. Tustison, N.J., et al.: Large-scale evaluation of ANTS and FreeSurfer cortical thickness measurements. Neuroimage **99**, 166–179 (2014)
20. Wang, G., Li, W., Ourselin, S., Vercauteren, T.: Automatic brain tumor segmentation using cascaded anisotropic convolutional neural networks. arXiv preprint arXiv:1709.00382 (2017)
21. Yang, D., et al.: Automatic liver segmentation using an adversarial image-to-image network. In: Descoteaux, M., Maier-Hein, L., Franz, A., Jannin, P., Collins, D.L., Duchesne, S. (eds.) MICCAI 2017 Part III. LNCS, vol. 10435, pp. 507–515. Springer, Cham (2017). https://doi.org/10.1007/978-3-319-66179-7_58
22. Zhang, Y., Yang, L., Chen, J., Fredericksen, M., Hughes, D.P., Chen, D.Z.: Deep adversarial networks for biomedical image segmentation utilizing unannotated images. In: Descoteaux, M., Maier-Hein, L., Franz, A., Jannin, P., Collins, D.L., Duchesne, S. (eds.) MICCAI 2017 Part III. LNCS, vol. 10435, pp. 408–416. Springer, Cham (2017). https://doi.org/10.1007/978-3-319-66179-7_47

Data Augmentation Using Synthetic Lesions Improves Machine Learning Detection of Microbleeds from MRI

Saba Momeni[1,2(✉)], Amir Fazllolahi[1], Pierrick Bourgeat[1],
Parnesh Raniga[1], Paul Yates[3], Nawaf Yassi[4], Patricia Desmond[4],
Jurgen Fripp[1], Yongsheng Gao[2], and Olivier Salvado[5]

[1] CSIRO Health and Biosecurity, Australian E-Health Research Centre,
Brisbane, Australia
saba.momeni@csiro.au
[2] Department of Engineering, Griffith University, Brisbane, Australia
[3] Department of Nuclear Medicine and Centre for PET,
Austin Health Heidelberg, Heidelberg, Australia
[4] University of Melbourne, Parkville, Australia
[5] Data61, Brisbane, Australia

Abstract. Machine learning applied to medical imaging for lesions detection, such as cerebral microbleeds (CMB) from Magnetic Resonance Imaging (MRI), is challenged by the relatively small datasets available for which only subjective and tedious visual reading is available, and by the low prevalence of lesions (a few in $\sim 10\%$ of a typical elderly cohort) resulting in unbalanced classes. Moreover, the lack of actual ground truth might limit the performance of any machine learning method to that of human performance. Yet, the automatic identification of those lesions is relevant to quantify cerebrovascular burden associated with dementia, such as identifying co-morbidity for Alzheimer's disease. In this paper, we investigated a novel approach consisting of simulating synthetic CMB on SWI MRI scans from healthy individuals to create a large and well characterized training dataset, as a data augmentation strategy. Firstly, we characterized actual CMBs from MRI SWI scans and designed a method to create realistic synthetic CMBs whose location, shape, appearance, and size are similar to actual CMBs. We then tested a supervised neural network classifier using various combinations of actual CMB and synthetic CMBs for training. Augmenting data with synthetic CMBs resulted in a large improvement over training on only actual CMBs only when tested on unseen lesions, and provided better results than other standard data augmentation approaches. Our results suggest that data augmentation using synthetic lesions can address the lack of ground truth and low prevalence limitations for medical imaging analysis allowing the deployment of data hungry supervised learning techniques such as deep learning.

Keywords: Cerebral microbleeds · Susceptibility weighted imaging
SWI · Machine learning · Data augmentation · Synthetic data

A. Gooya et al. (Eds.): SASHIMI 2018, LNCS 11037, pp. 12–19, 2018.
https://doi.org/10.1007/978-3-030-00536-8_2

1   Introduction

Cerebral microbleeds (CMBs) are hemosiderin deposit caused by structural abnormalities of the blood vessels [1]. They are prevalent in people suffering from cognitive and cerebrovascular disease such as stroke and Alzheimer's disease. They are also asymptomatic and present in cognitively normal individuals. The detection of CMB from MRI is thus clinically important to assess cerebrovascular burden.

Magnetic susceptibility is affected by the presence of CMB in brain parenchyma [2], and susceptibility-weighted imaging (SWI) [2] has been shown to image CMB with excellent sensitivity, limited mostly by the imaging resolution (typically $1 \times 1 \times 2$ mm^3). In SWI scans, CMBs appear as small spherical hypo-intense areas in tissue with a similar appearance than the numerous blood vessels, also seen in SWI, when observed in cross-section. For this reason, the clinical observation of CMB, often based on the Microbleed Anatomical Rating Scale (MARS) [3], is tedious and time-consuming because of the large number of similar features from blood vessels. Indeed, CMB mimics include vessel cross section, calcification, and cavernous malformation on SWI.

Automated methods are also challenged by the large number of mimics resulting in numerous false positives while there is a relatively small number of true positives since the prevalence is about a few CMB in 10% of asymptomatic elderly subjects [4]. This creates a large unbalance classes hampering supervised training, further compounded by the limited size of datasets where ground truth (human expert annotation) is available. To address this problem, data augmentation methods are often used [5]. Synthetic Minority Oversampling Technique SMOTE [5], is one strategy to balance the classes by generating new pseudo TP (true positives) instances from the existing minority TP cases. In this paper, we investigate data augmentation by generating synthetic CMBs. We compare this new approach to SMOTE and the other widely used data augmentation method using rotation and translation. We describe the method to create realistic synthetic CMB and demonstrate that performance of a neural network classifier can be improved by transferring the learning from the synthetic data to real clinical data. We do not aim at presenting a new classifier, but at demonstrating that using synthetic lesions can improve the performance of supervised learning. We use in this paper a simple feed forward Artificial Neural Network as a case example.

2   Method

2.1   Dataset

Data are from the Australian Imaging Biomarkers & Lifestyle (AIBL). We used 64 scans from 39 participants (including some repeat scans at 18 months interval). There were 24 patients clinically diagnosed with Alzheimer's disease (AD), 34 subjects with mild cognitive impairment (MCI) and 6 healthy controls (HC), with an average age of 79.21, 77.74 and 79.98, respectively. The scans comprised 27 females and 37 males. All subjects underwent an anatomical T1-weighted (T1 W) and a SWI acquisitions on a 3T Siemens TRIO scanner. SWI was reconstructed online using the scanner system (software VB17). The 3D SWI parameters were: 0.93×0.93 mm^2 in-plane resolution and 1.75 mm slice thickness, repetition time/echo time of 27/20 ms, and flip angle $20°$. T1 W images were acquired using a standard 3D magnetization-prepared rapid gradient echo (MPRAGE) sequence with in-plane resolution 1.0×1.0 mm^2, slice thickness 1.2 mm, repetition-time/echo-time/TI = 2.300/2.98/900, flip angle $9°$, field of view 240×256, and 160 slices. Scans were reviewed by two clinical experts and marked using the MARS criteria as definite and possible.

2.2   Preprocessing

For all the scans, N4 bias field correction technique [6], skull-stripping masking to exclude non-brain tissues [4], and histogram matching were applied before any processing. All SWI images were normalized between [0 1]. Brain tissues were segmented from the T1W into gray matter (GM), white matter (WM), and cerebrospinal fluid (CSF) using posterior probability classification after fitting a mixture of Gaussian distribution to the histogram using the expectation-minimization method. A final region of interest (ROI) mask was built by merging the WM and GM voxels.

2.3   Features of Actual CMBs

From the analysis of the SWI datasets, CMBs were characterized using four parameters: size, shape, intensity, and location. In our dataset, the CMBs were uniformly located in the WM, GM tissues, and therefore location of synthetic lesions was uniformly distributed in the corresponding mask.

CMB Intensity: It was observed that large CMB intensity had a minimum value of 0, while the intensity of smaller size lesions became closer to tissue intensity. Figure 1 top left panel shows the minimum value of expert identified CMB. We assumed that this effect was entirely due to partial volume effect and that the minimum intensity value of a CMB is 0. This is consistent with SWI processing where the square of the high frequency filtered phase multiplies the signal magnitude, resulting in 0 intensity.

CMB Size: $11 \times 11 \times 11$ patches with definite CMB at their center were extracted from the 64 SWI images, resulting in 144 patches making up the TP class. For each patch, a mixture of distributions was fitted using the expectation minimization algorithm: a Gaussian to model brain tissues and a uniform distribution to model outliers due to partial volume effect, and low intensity pixels from vessels and CMBs. A maximum a posterior classification was performed to create a mask of the CMB in the patch (cleaned using connected components). The mean of the Gaussian was assumed to be the tissue mean intensity while an intensity of zero was assumed to be the intensity of the CMB. Fractional CMB content was estimated for each pixel of the CMB mask by using a standard partial volume model. Eventually, fractions of CMB for each pixel were summed up to estimate the volume of each CMB as shown in Fig. 1.

2.4   Generation of Synthetic CMBs

It is our goal to create realistic synthetic CMB (sCMB), which should thus have the same characteristics as the real ones defined in the previous section.

A 3D Gaussian function was generated on a $110 \times 110 \times 110$ patch (ratio matching the SWI resolution ratio). Its location was the center of the middle pixel of the patch with added uniform random noise in all three axis within $[\pm 15, \pm 15, \pm 15]$ voxels. In order to simulate variation around a spherical shape, given a spherical volume, two of the 3D Gaussian standard deviations were multiplied by a random number between 0.5 and 0.9, while the third one was defined so that the overall volume was conserved. The shape was adjusted using the 3D Gaussian standard deviations to match the actual SWI resolution ratio. Random variation of the three standard deviation values of the 3D Gaussian allowed random variation of shape around a mean ellipsoid while keeping the same overall volume. The volume of the sCMB was randomly sampled from a smooth approximation of the size distribution of real CMBs (shown in Fig. 1 top left panel). Uniform random rotation was also added on the three axis within $\pm 30°$.

The Gaussian intensity profile was thresholded at half maximum to create a mask simulating a high resolution sCMB (0 within the mask and 1 outside). The patch was then down sampled to $11 \times 11 \times 11$ to simulate partial volume effect (values ranging between 0 and 1 to simulate PVE). The resulting patches were then multiplied with patches extracted from the SWI images without any CMB, whose selection is explained in the next section. As a results, a synthetic TP patch (sTP) could be created for which the lesion size and appearance could be computed in the same way as actual CMB patches as explained in the previous section and displayed in Fig. 1 right panels.

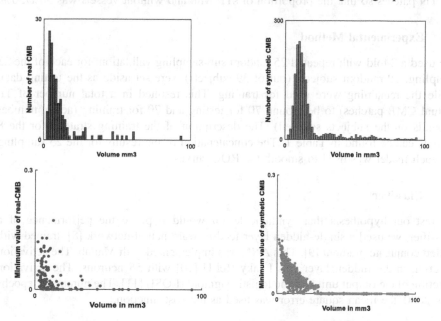

Fig. 1. The size distribution (top panels) and minimum intensity (bottom panels) for the real CMB in blue (left panels) and the generated synthetic CMB in red (right panels). The minimum intensities are comparable and entirely due to partial volume effect in the synthetic case. (Color figure online)

Table 1. Models considered in this study with approximate number of patches in each class.

Model	# of TP	# of sTP	# of TN	Comment
M1	70	0	140	Train on actual only
M2	70	0	1400	M1 but highly unbalanced
M3	70	1200	1400	Train on actual + synthetic
M4	0	1200	1400	Train only on Synthetic
M5	0	70	140	Train on synthetic with same size as M1
M6	70	1200	1400	Train on augmented data
M7	70	600 + 600	1400	Train on synthetic + augmented data
M8	70	1200	1400	Train on augmented data by SMOTE [5]

2.5 Patch Extraction

From the SWI dataset, patches were extracted and assigned to two categories: (1) Patches with real CMB defined as definite by the two experts (TP), (2) Patches with no actual CMB (neither definite nor possible). The second type was further divided into those patches containing either blood vessels or some CSF (seen as dark and possibly confounding CMB), and patches containing mostly GM or WM tissues. They were labeled as true negative (TN) with and without blood vessels. Vessels were detected using the Radial Symmetry Transform RST [7]. In order to create a patch with a synthetic CMB, the $11 \times 11 \times 11$ mask described in the previous section was multiplied with a patch from the TN class, creating a synthetic TP patch (sTP). We selected the TN patches so that the proportion of sTP with and without vessels was 50%/50%.

2.6 Experimental Method

We used a 2-fold with repeated 25 random sub-sampling validation: for each of the 25 sampling, 19 random subjects (out of 39 subjects) were set aside as the testing data, while the remaining were used for training. This resulted in a total number of TP (actual CMB patches) to be around 70 for testing and 70 for training (actual number depends on the subjects selected). The description of the training strategy for the 8 models can be found in Table 1. The concatenation of the results for the 25 sampling for each model was used to smooth the ROC curves.

2.7 Classifier

To test our hypothesis that synthetic lesion would improve the performance of a classifier, we used a single-hidden layer feed-forward neural-network [8], trained with scaled conjugate gradient [9]. This ANN was implemented with Matlab. The activation function in the hidden layer was Leaky ReLU [10] with 55 neurons. The activation function of the output unit was the logistic sigmoid (LOSI) [11]. The number of epochs was 2000, the mean square error was used as the cost function.

Real CMB (TP)   Synthetic CMB (sTP)   TN with vessel   TN without vessel

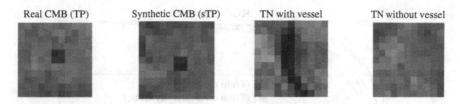

Fig. 2. Typical examples of axial section for the different classes. Note that the sCMB is not centered (second left panel), similar to the real one (left panel), because we added random variation in location and shape.

3   Results and Discussion

3.1   Synthetic CMB Generation

Synthetic CMB could be created with no discernable differences from actual lesions. The size and intensity were similar between actual and synthetic lesions as shown in Fig. 1. The location of synthetic samples was uniform in the GM and WM tissues as observed for real ones. Figure 2 shows examples of axial sections from the $11 \times 11 \times 11$ patches.

3.2   Results of CMB Classification Using ANN

Results for the ANN classification on the testing datasets is reported in Table 2. We show the area under ROC (AUR), mean sensitivity, specificity and accuracy along with the standard deviation over the 25 sampling 2-fold cross validation design. Model 2 would not converge to any meaningful results due to the unbalanced classes and is omitted here. Figure 3 shows the ROC curve for all the models. The results using SMOTE (model 8) were the lowest of the three data augmentation methods. Using synthetic data provided good results, and the best model was the one training on synthetic data alone. Merging synthetic with the TP class had also good results close to training on synthetic data alone. Using standard geometric data augmentation improved performance but not as much strategy involving using synthetic data.

Table 2. Performance of the models on the test datasets. Values are averages ± standard deviation over the 25 draws from averaging the outputs. Bold shows the best performance models.

Model	Accuracy	Sensitivity	Specificity	AUR
M1	0.88 ± 0.022	0.87 ± 0.028	0.88 ± 0.030	0.93 ± 0.020
M3	**0.91 ± 0.021**	**0.90 ± 0.035**	**0.91 ± 0.026**	**0.95 ± 0.018**
M4	0.90 ± 0.021	**0.90 ± 0.029**	**0.91 ± 0.030**	**0.95 ± 0.018**
M5	0.83 ± 0.033	0.85 ± 0.037	0.82 ± 0.050	0.89 ± 0.024
M6	0.88 ± 0.014	0.87 ± 0.035	0.88 ± 0.024	0.93 ± 0.012
M7	0.90 ± 0.019	0.89 ± 0.034	**0.91 ± 0.026**	**0.95 ± 0.013**
M8	0.85 ± 0.020	0.87 ± 0.032	0.84 ± 0.031	0.91 ± 0.016

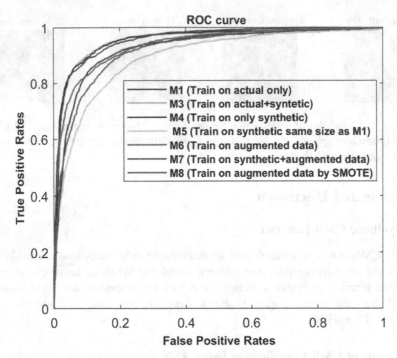

Fig. 3. ROC curve for the different models using a 2-fold with repeated 25 random sub-sampling validation design.

3.3 Discussion

Our results suggest that augmenting data with synthetic lesions could help increasing supervised classifier performance to detect microbleeds in MRI SWI. The best results were obtained by training on synthetic data alone even though the performance were measured on real data.

Our proposed approach addresses one critical issue for lesion detection task: when the prevalence of a lesion type is low, a very small number of TP are available for training supervised classifier limiting the complexity of the possible models to consider. Another consequence is the class unbalanced between the positive and negative. Indeed, the naïve approach of training the ANN on very unbalanced data (1:10) failed to produce any meaningful results. Adding sCMB allowed to balance the classes and increased the number of examples resulting in much improved performance.

Our proposed approach is very dependent on how realistic the synthetic lesions are created. We described a simple method based on a Gaussian profile that is added to the magnitude SWI images (magnitude multiplied by filtered phase). A better characterization of actual microbleeds using high resolution MRI, such as 7T, could help improve the generation of simulated lesions. In addition, adding the synthetic lesions on the complex image, before SWI processing, might improve the realism of the synthetic data.

Despite those limitations, augmenting medical data using synthetic lesions could allow to use complex classifiers, such as deep learning network, with large number of parameters since arbitrary large training datasets could be created along with the perfect ground truth necessary for supervised learning. Of course that approach is limited by how close the synthetic ground truth is from the actual and elusive ground truth. This is tantamount to converting human expertise (a priori knowledge about what lesions look like) into data that is then transfer through learning into the weights of a classifier. More research on different applications would inform whether our proposed approach could allow automated methods to push performance beyond that of experts.

References

1. Martinez-Ramirez, S., Greenberg, S.M., Viswanathan, A.: Cerebral microbleeds: overview and implications in cognitive impairment. Alzheimers Res. Ther. **6**(3), 33 (2014)
2. Haacke, E.M., Mittal, S., Wu, Z., Neelavalli, J., Cheng, Y.-C.N.: Susceptibility-weighted imaging: technical aspects and clinical applications, part 1. Am. J. Neuroradiol. **30**(1), 19–30 (2009)
3. The Microbleed Anatomical Rating Scale (MARS) | Neurology. http://n.neurology.org/content/73/21/1759. Accessed 30 Apr 2018
4. Fazlollahi, A., et al.: Computer-aided detection of cerebral microbleeds in susceptibility-weighted imaging. Comput. Med. Imaging Graph. **46**(Part 3), 269–276 (2015)
5. He, H., Garcia, E.A.: Learning from imbalanced data. IEEE Trans. Knowl. Data Eng. **21**(9), 1263–1284 (2009)
6. Tustison, N.J., et al.: N4ITK: improved N3 bias correction. IEEE Trans. Med. Imaging **29**(6), 1310–1320 (2010)
7. Loy, G., Zelinsky, A.: Fast radial symmetry for detecting points of interest. IEEE Trans. Pattern Anal. Mach. Intell. **25**(8), 959–973 (2003)
8. Bin, L., Xuewen, R.: Review and performance analysis of single hidden layer sequential learning algorithms of feed-forward neural networks. In: 2013 25th Chinese Control and Decision Conference, CCDC 2013, pp. 2170–2175 (2013)
9. Livieris, I.E., Pintelas, P.: A new conjugate gradient algorithm for training neural networks based on a modified secant equation. Appl. Math. Comput. **221**, 491–502 (2013)
10. Aghdam, H.H., Heravi, E.J., Puig, D.: Recognizing traffic signs using a practical deep neural network. Robot 2015: Second Iberian Robotics Conference. AISC, vol. 417, pp. 399–410. Springer, Cham (2016). https://doi.org/10.1007/978-3-319-27146-0_31
11. Zadeh, M.R., Amin, S., Khalili, D., Singh, V.P.: Daily outflow prediction by multi layer perceptron with logistic sigmoid and tangent sigmoid activation functions. Water Resour. Manag. **24**(11), 2673–2688 (2010)

Deep Harmonization of Inconsistent MR Data for Consistent Volume Segmentation

Blake E. Dewey[1,2(✉)], Can Zhao[1], Aaron Carass[1], Jiwon Oh[3],
Peter A. Calabresi[3], Peter C. M. van Zijl[2,4], and Jerry L. Prince[1,4]

[1] Department of Electrical and Computer Engineering,
The Johns Hopkins University, Baltimore, MD, USA
blake.dewey@jhu.edu
[2] Kirby Center for Functional Brain Imaging,
Kennedy Krieger Institute, Baltimore, MD, USA
[3] Department of Neurology,
The Johns Hopkins School of Medicine, Baltimore, MD, USA
[4] Department of Radiology and Radiological Science,
The Johns Hopkins School of Medicine, Baltimore, MD, USA

Abstract. Magnetic resonance image analysis is often hampered by inconsistent data due to upgrades or changes to the scanner platform or modification of scanning protocols. These changes can manifest in three main sources of image inconsistency: contrast, resolution, and noise. Modern analysis techniques that use supervised machine learning can be especially susceptible to these inconsistencies, as existing training data may not be valid after an upgrade or protocol change. In previous work, differences in contrast and resolution have been addressed in isolation. We propose a novel method of image intensity harmonization that addresses each of the three sources of inconsistency. We formulate our method around a multi-planar, multi-contrast U-net, where all of the available contrasts are used as input channels in a single modified U-Net to produce all of the output contrasts simultaneously. The multi-contrast nature of the deep network allows for harmonization of contrast as information can be shared between contrasts. In addition, coherent, biological features are highlighted and matched to the target, while noise, which differs between matched inputs and outputs, is not reinforced. This process also normalizes small differences in resolution due to the influence of the high resolution channels. To combat larger differences in resolution, which would not be recovered by the neural network alone, we use self super-resolution (SSR) on all images with thick (>2 mm) slices before harmonization. To generate consistent images, the target images are also processed in a similar manner so that all resulting images have consistent qualities. Our harmonization process eliminates significant volume bias of multiple brain compartments and lesion estimation. In addition, absolute volume difference and Dice similarity of segmentation volumes were significantly improved ($p < 0.005$). SSR alone did not affect the statistical significance of the difference, even though the absolute volume difference was reduced.

© Springer Nature Switzerland AG 2018
A. Gooya et al. (Eds.): SASHIMI 2018, LNCS 11037, pp. 20–30, 2018.
https://doi.org/10.1007/978-3-030-00536-8_3

Keywords: MR harmonization · Super-resolution
Multiple sclerosis · Deep learning

1   Introduction

Magnetic resonance imaging (MRI) is a non-invasive medical imaging technique often used to image the brain due to the high contrast in soft tissue and low contribution of signal from bone. However, structural images in MRI are not quantitative, but instead have arbitrary units that are driven by the "weight" of the image. For example, a "T1-weighted" image has contrast that is primarily driven by the longitudinal relaxation time, T1. The method of acquisition for T1-weighted imaging, however, varies greatly between sites and vendors. Differences in scanner manufacturer, scanner hardware, or even scanner software can cause detrimental intra- and inter-site variation, particularly if upgrades or protocol changes occur during a study [13]. This is an ubiquitous problem, especially in multi-site or longitudinal studies, where consistent imaging has been found to be nearly impossible. We aim to achieve stable, consistent automated analyses by harmonizing the input images with respect to three interdependent sources of inconsistency: contrast, noise, and resolution.

Magnetic Resonance (MR) image harmonization has been previously addressed in different ways. The simplest methods modify intensities to normalize the histograms of the input images, either in a linear or piecewise manner [8]. These methods benefit from being globally applicable, but they capture no information about the spatial aspects of contrast and can be shown to produce highly inconsistent results [6]. Other methods tackle contrast specifically using patch-based approaches to match contrast intensities by incorporating spatial information of the local area [9,11]. These methods require preprocessing steps such as skull-stripping to perform properly, as the small patch methods that are used are not capable of distinguishing between extra-cerebral tissue that matches intensities on a local scale with brain tissue. Previous methods also do not take into account multiple sources of inconsistency, and instead focus on contrast [7,11] or resolution [9] individually. In addition, all previous methods only incorporate information from one 2D orientation (or a very restricted 3D patch), restricting information from other planes. This is a severe limitation when using harmonization for consistent segmentation, as segmented structures are defined in 3D.

Recently, attempts have been made to incorporate convolutional neural networks (CNN) to synthesize new image contrasts [4,17]. We propose a novel CNN-based harmonization method for image normalization that incorporates multi-contrast and multi-planar information to produce highly similar structural images for consistent image segmentation. To do this, we build on existing methods by incorporating multi-contrast information into a U-net modified for improved synthesis results [17]. However, unlike the work done by Chartsias et al. [4], multi-contrast information is used within a single trained network to allow for maximum cross-utilization of different contrast information. Our network is

Table 1. Scanner and protocol specifications

	Scanner #1	Scanner #2
Scanner hardware	Philips Achieva 3T	Philips Achieva 3T
Scanner software	R3.2.3	R5.1.7
Receive coil	16ch Neurovascular	32ch Head
T1-weighted	MPRAGE	MEMPRAGE
	$1.1 \times 1.1 \times 1.18$ mm*	$1 \times 1 \times 1$ mm
	TE $= 6$ ms, TR $= 3$ s, TI $= 840$ ms	TE $= 6.2$ ms, TR $= 2.5$ s, TI $= 900$ ms
FLAIR	2D TSE	3D VISTA (TSE)
	$0.83 \times 0.83 \times 2.2$ mm	$1 \times 1 \times 1$ mm
	TE $= 68$ ms, TR $= 11$ s, TI $= 2.8$ s	TE $= 125$ ms, TR $= 4.8$ s, TI $= 1.6$ s
PD-/T2-weighted	2D TSE	2D TSE
	$1.1 \times 1.1 \times 2.2$ mm*	$1 \times 1 \times 3$ mm
	TE $= 12$ ms/80 ms, TR $= 4.2$ s	TE $= 11$ ms/100 ms, TR $= 3.4$ s

*Scan is reconstructed on the scanner 0.83×0.83 mm in-plane by zero-padding in frequency space

additionally trained and applied in three orthogonal directions to maximize the ability for resolution recovery in low resolution images and minimize the effect of artifacts during the harmonization process, especially slice-to-slice differences. We also compare the effectiveness of self super-resolution (SSR) alone in lesion and intracranial volume segmentation to account for large changes in resolution, while ignoring changes in contrast.

2 Methods

2.1 Image Acquisition/Preprocessing

MR images were acquired using two different Philips Achieva 3T scanners with different major release software versions. Healthy controls (HC) ($n = 2$) and multiple sclerosis (MS) patients ($n = 10$) were recruited under a local Institutional Review Board protocol and provided informed consent. Each subject underwent a research scanning protocol on each scanner less than one month apart. Scanner and protocols specifications for each of the two acquisition methods are outlined in Table 1 with example images in Fig. 1. The time to acquire all images was 12:45 min for Scanner #1 and 15:15 min for Scanner #2. All images were reoriented to axial orientation, corrected for inhomogeneity with N4 Bias Correction [14], and normalized to the white matter peak (WMP). SSR was also performed on all images with thick (>2 mm) slices using the SMORE [16] technique. SMORE uses multiple EDSR super-resolution networks to perform

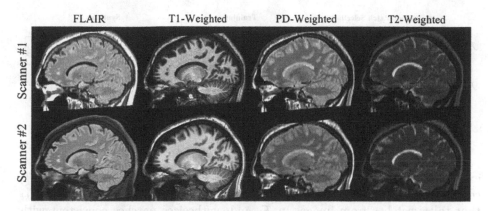

Fig. 1. Example images from Scanner #1 (top row) and Scanner #2 (bottom row) for a single subject. All images have been co-registered and white matter peak normalized to highlight contrast differences. The same display window is used for all images.

anti-aliasing and SSR sequentially, allowing for increased accuracy in images with thicker slices. All thick slice, N4-corrected images for each subject were passed into the online training process for both SMORE networks with a set of pre-trained weights that were trained on similar images. Final weights from online training were applied to each of the low resolution directions and a final image was created via Fourier burst accumulation [5]. Rigid co-registration within subjects was performed for each subject with additional rigid registration between subjects using Advanced Normalization Tools [1]. The final images were created by B-spline interpolation using a combined transformation. To compare the effect of different normalization pipelines, the original images after N4 correction were also transformed to create a separate set of baseline images where only WMP normalization was used (termed WMP). 3D isotropic (or near isotropic images) will be identical in these two sets, as SSR was only performed on images with thick slices.

2.2 CNN Harmonization

Let $\mathbf{f}_k^i = \left\{ f_k^{i,1}, \ldots, f_k^{i,C_k} \right\}$ be a set of co-registered, preprocessed images acquired during a single scanning session on scanner k, where C_k is the number of contrasts acquired. In general, we have a collection of image sets $\mathcal{F}_k = \left\{ \mathbf{f}_k^i \right\}_{i=1\ldots N_k}$, which have been acquired on scanner k, that we would like to normalize to images $\mathcal{F}_l$ acquired on scanner l. In this paper, k and l are both drawn from $\{1,2\}$ as only two scanners are considered. For training, we acquire a prospective subset on each scanner, $\mathcal{F}_{k,l}^n = \left\{ \mathbf{f}_{k,l}^i \right\}_{i=1\ldots n}$, such that, for all $i = 1, \ldots, n$, $\{\mathbf{f}_1^i, \mathbf{f}_k^i\}$ come from the same patient within a short time frame (≤ 1 month). From $\mathcal{F}_k^n$, we

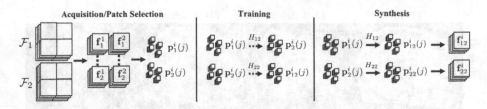

Fig. 2. Diagram outlining CNN harmonization.

extract patches $\mathbf{p}_k^i(j)$ such that $\mathbf{p}_k^i(j)$ is a $128 \times 128 \times C_k$ patch from image $\mathbf{f}_k^i$, centered at voxel j. We represent our CNN-based synthesis as an operator H_{kl} that takes patches from images in $\mathcal{F}_k$ and synthesizes patches consistent with images from scanner l ($H_{kl} : \mathbf{p}_k^i(j) \to \widehat{\mathbf{p}}_{kl}^i(j)$). To train H_{kl}, we randomly select $\mathbf{p}_k^i(j)$ from $\mathcal{F}_k^n$ as inputs and evaluate against the corresponding patches $\mathbf{p}_l^i(j)$ from $\mathcal{F}_l^n$ centered at the same center voxel j. In the special case of H_{ll}, synthetic data created from the other scanner ($\widehat{\mathbf{p}}_{kl}^i(j)$) is used as the target data to avoid an identity transform. In the testing phase, a sliding window is used to select $\mathbf{p}_k^i(j)$ to cover the entire image $\mathbf{f}_k^i(j)$ and H_{kl} is applied to create the synthetic patches $\widehat{\mathbf{p}}_{kl}^i(j)$. The final synthetic image $\widehat{\mathbf{f}}_{kl}^i$ is generated by taking the mean of all overlapping estimated patches at each voxel. This process is also briefly explained in Fig. 2.

To reduce artifacts and incorporate multi-planar information in the final images, three separate instances of H_{kl} are trained for each scanner by reorienting the input and target images into each of the orthogonal planes (axial, sagittal, and coronal). For prediction, patches are extracted from the reoriented images and passed through the corresponding network (axial, sagittal, or coronal) and a direction-specific synthetic image is created. To create the final (multi-planer) synthetic image, the voxel-wise median is calculated from these three direction-specific images.

For this study, all instances of H_{kl} were constructed using a 2D U-net that was modified for synthesis by adding a skip connection between the input images and the final feature maps, as described in [17]. The network and training were designed in Keras using TensorFlow as the underlying deep learning library. Input patches of 128×128 voxels were selected randomly for training. Each network was trained for 100 epochs of 250 batches (batch size of 32) using the ADAM optimizer and a learning rate of 0.001 and training time was approximately 8 h on an NVIDIA Tesla K80. To separate training and testing data, the available training data was split into two groups of 6 subjects (1 HC and 5 MS) and testing for images in each group was performed using weights trained on the other group to preserve training/testing separation. Scanner #2 was selected as the target during training, as the images represent the current state of the art for structural imaging and provide superior gray matter/white matter and lesion contrast. In theory, the method could be trained and applied in the opposite direction, but the final images, while being normalized between the two scanners, would take on the inferior qualities of the Scanner #1 images.

After training of H_{kl} was completed, all training images from scanner k were passed through H_{kl} to create a training set for H_{ll}. In the case of greater than 2 scanners to be normalized, all scanners $\{k\}_{k \neq l}$ will be processed in this way to create a singular training set for H_{ll}. The training of H_{ll} is a vital step to the harmonization process that allows for all final images to have the qualities of the synthetic images. Without this network, the images from scanner l would have the native image features (especially noise), which would greatly differ from the harmonized images from scanner l. Therefore, we use H_{ll} to harmonize the scanner l images into the same image domain.

2.3   Analysis Pipeline

After synthesis, standard post-processing and segmentation methods were performed. Skull removal was performed using MONSTR [10]. The resulting mask also served as an estimate of intracranial volume (ICV). The skull-stripped images were then used for further volumetric analysis. For the 10 MS subjects, white matter lesion (WML) segmentation was performed using a multi-view CNN segmentation routine [2], with the T1-weighted and corresponding FLAIR images as inputs. Training for this network was performed on training data from the ISBI 2015 White Matter Lesion Segmentation Challenge [3]. To remove false positives, a WML-inclusive WM mask was created using LesionTOADS [12] and applied to the CNN segmentation. Whole brain segmentation was also performed using Joint Label Fusion (JLF) [15]. To properly segment the brains with WML, the lesion mask was also used to fill the T1-weighted images using the lesion_filling tool from FSL before JLF.

After segmentation, anatomical volumes were calculated and compared between scanners for each of the three normalization pipelines (WMP baseline, SSR only, and SSR with CNN-based harmonization). In addition to the comparison of volume measurements directly using absolute percent volume difference and signed volume difference (volume bias), Dice similarity coefficient (DSC) between scanners were also calculated. The resulting harmonized images from each of the three pipelines were also evaluated for similarity and quality using structured similarity (SSIM) and mean squared error (MSE). All statistical tests were performed using the Wilcoxon signed-rank test and statistical significance was determined at the $\alpha = 0.005$ level.

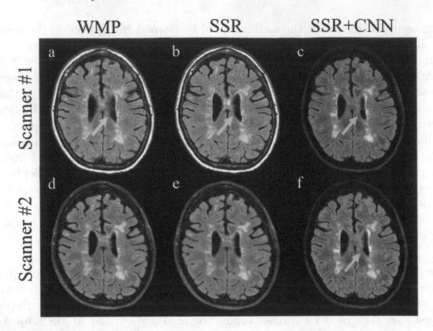

Fig. 3. Results from WMP normalization (a, d), SSR (b, e) and SSR with CNN harmonization (c, f) on FLAIR images from Scanner 1 (a, b, c) and Scanner 2 (d, e, f). Red arrows show differences in ventricles between scanners, while green arrows show similarities in SSR + CNN synthesized images. The same intensity windowing is used for all images. (Color figure online)

3   Results

Qualitative results of each processing pipeline are shown in Figs. 3 and 4. The harmonized images (Figs. 3(c, f) and 4(b, d)) have qualitative consistency in intensity, as well as a recovery of apparent resolution in the low resolution directions of the 2D-acquired images (FLAIR, PD-weighted, and T2-weighted). This is especially evident in the FLAIR images (Fig. 3), where the ventricles are poorly defined

Table 2. Volume bias (in %) between Scanner #1 and Scanner #2 after different normalization pipelines. Bold values indicate the the bias is significant when compared to 0.

	WMP	SSR	SSR + CNN
Cortical GM	−0.529	−0.491	−0.392
Cerebral WM	**2.631**	**2.740**	0.350
Cerebellar GM	**−6.097**	**−5.293**	−0.078
Cerebellar WM	**−5.331**	**−5.176**	−2.103
Thalamus	1.607	1.601	−0.390
Lateral ventricle	**−6.484**	**−6.663**	0.104
ICV	**−0.542**	**−0.330**	−0.235
WML	**−18.862**	**−11.801**	4.216

in the Scanner #1 acquisitions (Fig. 3(a)). They are more precisely defined in the harmonized version of Scanner #1 (Fig. 3(c)). As is expected from the qualitative results, the addition of CNN harmonization greatly improves image sim-

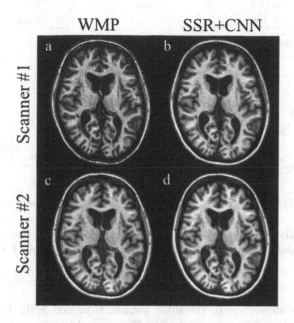

Fig. 4. Results of each normalization pipeline on T1-weighted images. SSR is not included as SSR was not performed independently on T1-weighted images. For the SSR + CNN, result all thick slice input images were preprocessed with SSR. The same windowing is used for all images.

Table 3. Mean (standard deviation) overlap and volume measures for whole-brain and lesion segmentation results

	Dice similarity			% Volume difference		
	WMP	SSR	CNN + SSR	WMP	SSR	CNN + SSR
Cortical GM	0.917 (0.015)	0.916 (0.015)	**0.951 (0.017)**	1.998 (1.134)	2.118 (1.271)	**0.790 (0.988)**
Cerebral WM	0.954 (0.007)	0.953 (0.007)	**0.964 (0.006)**	2.510 (1.441)	2.611 (1.503)	**0.879 (0.800)**
Cerebellar GM	0.934 (0.008)	0.936 (0.008)	**0.967 (0.005)**	5.457 (2.045)	6.239 (2.300)	**1.333 (1.008)**
Cerebellar WM	0.942 (0.022)	0.942 (0.022)	0.954 (0.011)	4.945 (5.563)	4.992 (5.567)	**2.815 (2.202)**
Thalamus	0.960 (0.006)	0.960 (0.006)	0.960 (0.006)	2.186 (1.671)	2.209 (1.697)	2.996 (1.842)
Lateral Ventricle	0.956 (0.012)	0.955 (0.013)	**0.974 (0.007)**	6.298 (1.981)	6.471 (2.110)	**0.911 (0.645)**
ICV	0.986 (0.003)	0.986 (0.004)	**0.990 (0.007)**	0.671 (0.478)	0.694 (0.507)	**0.756 (0.529)**
WML	0.708 (0.120)	0.705 (0.105)	**0.805 (0.060)**	18.86 (14.09)	**13.14 (7.753)**	9.582 (5.754)

Note: Bold indicates significant difference with respect to WMP.

ilarity and consistency in all measured metrics. In Fig. 5, we show substantial and significant improvements in SSIM (Fig. 5(a)) and MSE (Fig. 5(b)) after the inclusion of CNN-based harmonization, when compared to either the WMP or SSR normalized images.

In the comparison of automated segmentations, all investigated volumes (except cortical GM and thalamus) showed a significant bias between Scanner #1 and Scanner #2 when only WMP normalization was used. This persisted with the introduction of SSR, which is expected as the T1 images did not undergo any

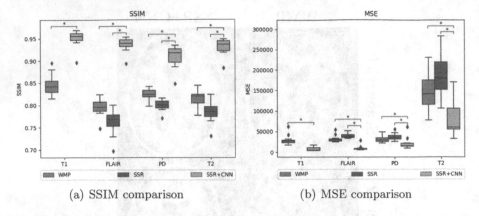

(a) SSIM comparison   (b) MSE comparison

Fig. 5. Quantitative comparison of skull-stripped volumes after each normalization pipeline. Statistical significance for each experiment is compared to CNN + SSR (*p < 0.005).

SSR beyond the difference in the filled lesions. However, SSR did significantly improve the volume difference in the WML class, which depends highly on the FLAIR image, which benefits from SSR. After CNN-based harmonization, no significant difference was found in any compartment. These data are reported in Table 2. In addition to the reduction of statistical bias in quantitative volumes, there are substantial differences in DSC and percent volume difference when compared to the WMP baseline. Specific values are provided in Table 3. For volume estimates, reductions in absolute difference between scanners of 2–5 times were observed in larger structures (cortical GM, cerebral WM, cerebellar GM, cerebellar WM, and lateral ventricles), with all differences being significant except for the thalamus. When comparing the overlap of segmentations, the DSC values of CNN harmonized results were significantly increased in all compartments except for the Cerebellar WM and thalamus. Absolute volume difference between scanners after WMP and SSR methods was significantly reduced when compared to CNN + SSR in all areas except that of the thalamus. There was no significant difference between the WMP and SSR techniques.

4   Discussion and Conclusion

This paper presents a novel approach to MR image intensity harmonization through the use of multi-contrast and multi-planar CNN-based deep learning. In addition, we examined the use of SSR as an additional method to overcome large differences in resolution, while ignoring changes in contrast. We show that the quantitative similarity in image contrast and segmentation metrics is significantly improved with the addition of CNN-based harmonization. We note that the true benefits of SSR may only be realized in clinical images, which typically have larger slice thicknesses (as large as 4 or 5 mm) than the research images studied here. While we are unable to validate against a ground truth to determine accuracy, these results demonstrate that by acquiring a small cohort of overlapping subjects between scanner changes, our multi-planar, multi-contrast CNN can create images of consistent quality and produce comparable segmentation results between scanners. This will allow for continuous study of longitudinal cohorts where scanner changes are often inevitable and preclude accurate assessment of changes over time.

Acknowledgements. This research was supported by NIH grants R01NS082347 and P41EB015909, as well as a grant from the National Multiple Sclerosis Society (RG-1601-07180).

References

1. Avants, B.B., Tustison, N.J., Stauffer, M., Song, G., Wu, B., Gee, J.C.: The insight toolkit image registration framework. Front. Neuroinformatics **8**, 44 (2014)
2. Birenbaum, A., Greenspan, H.: Multi-view longitudinal CNN for multiple sclerosis lesion segmentation. Eng. Appl. Artif. Intell. **65**, 111–118 (2017)
3. Carass, A., et al.: Longitudinal multiple sclerosis lesion segmentation: resource and challenge. NeuroImage **148**, 77–102 (2017)
4. Chartsias, A., Joyce, T., Giuffrida, M.V., Tsaftaris, S.A.: Multimodal MR synthesis via modality-invariant latent representation. IEEE Trans. Med. Imaging **37**(3), 1–814 (2017)
5. Delbracio, M., Sapiro, G.: Removing camera shake via weighted fourier burst accumulation. IEEE Trans. Image Process. **24**(11), 3293–3307 (2015)
6. Fortin, J.P., Sweeney, E.M., Muschelli, J., Crainiceanu, C.M., Shinohara, R.T.: Alzheimers disease neuroimaging initiative: removing inter-subject technical variability in magnetic resonance imaging studies. Neuroimage **132**, 198–212 (2016)
7. Jog, A., Carass, A., Roy, S., Pham, D.L., Prince, J.L.: Random forest regression for magnetic resonance image synthesis. Med. Image Anal. **35**, 475–488 (2017)
8. Nyúl, L.G., Udupa, J.K., Zhang, X.: New variants of a method of MRI scale standardization. IEEE Trans. Med. Imaging **19**(2), 143–150 (2000)
9. Rousseau, F.: Brain hallucination. In: Forsyth, D., Torr, P., Zisserman, A. (eds.) ECCV 2008. LNCS, vol. 5302, pp. 497–508. Springer, Heidelberg (2008). https://doi.org/10.1007/978-3-540-88682-2_38
10. Roy, S., Butman, J.A., Pham, D.L.: Alzheimers disease neuroimaging initiative: robust skull stripping using multiple MR image contrasts insensitive to pathology. Neuroimage **146**, 132–147 (2017)
11. Roy, S., Carass, A., Prince, J.: A compressed sensing approach for MR tissue contrast synthesis. In: Székely, G., Hahn, H.K. (eds.) IPMI 2011. LNCS, vol. 6801, pp. 371–383. Springer, Heidelberg (2011). https://doi.org/10.1007/978-3-642-22092-0_31
12. Shiee, N., Bazin, P.L., Ozturk, A., Reich, D.S., Calabresi, P.A., Pham, D.L.: A topology-preserving approach to the segmentation of brain images with multiple sclerosis lesions. Neuroimage **49**(2), 1524–1535 (2010)
13. Shinohara, R.T., et al.: Volumetric analysis from a harmonized multisite brain MRI study of a single subject with multiple sclerosis. Am. J. Neuroradiol. **38**(8), 1501–1509 (2017)

14. Tustison, N.J., et al.: N4ITK: improved N3 bias correction. IEEE Trans. Med. Imaging **29**(6), 1310–1320 (2010)
15. Wang, H., Suh, J.W., Das, S.R., Pluta, J., Craige, C., Yushkevich, P.A.: Multi-atlas segmentation with joint label fusion. IEEE Trans. Pattern Anal. Mach. Intell. **35**(3), 611–623 (2013)
16. Zhao, C., et al.: A deep learning based anti-aliasing self super-resolution algorithm for MRI. In: 21st International Conference on Medical Image Computing and Computer-Assisted Intervention – MICCAI 2018. Springer (2018)
17. Zhao, C., Carass, A., Lee, J., He, Y., Prince, J.L.: Whole brain segmentation and labeling from CT using synthetic MR images. In: Wang, Q., Shi, Y., Suk, H.-I., Suzuki, K. (eds.) MLMI 2017. LNCS, vol. 10541, pp. 291–298. Springer, Cham (2017). https://doi.org/10.1007/978-3-319-67389-9_34

Cross-Modality Image Synthesis from Unpaired Data Using CycleGAN
Effects of Gradient Consistency Loss and Training Data Size

Yuta Hiasa[1](✉), Yoshito Otake[1], Masaki Takao[2], Takumi Matsuoka[1],
Kazuma Takashima[2], Aaron Carass[3], Jerry L. Prince[3], Nobuhiko Sugano[2],
and Yoshinobu Sato[1]

[1] Graduate School of Science and Technology,
Nara Institute of Science and Technology,
8916-5, Takayamacho, Ikomashi, Nara 630-0192, Japan
hiasa.yuta.ht7@is.naist.jp
[2] Graduate School of Medicine, Osaka University, Suita, Japan
[3] Department of Electrical and Computer Engineering,
Johns Hopkins University, Baltimore, USA

Abstract. CT is commonly used in orthopedic procedures. MRI is used
along with CT to identify muscle structures and diagnose osteonecrosis
due to its superior soft tissue contrast. However, MRI has poor contrast
for bone structures. Clearly, it would be helpful if a corresponding CT
were available, as bone boundaries are more clearly seen and CT has
a standardized (i.e., Hounsfield) unit. Therefore, we aim at MR-to-CT
synthesis. While the CycleGAN was successfully applied to unpaired CT
and MR images of the head, these images do not have as much variation
of intensity pairs as do images in the pelvic region due to the presence
of joints and muscles. In this paper, we extended the CycleGAN approach by adding the gradient consistency loss to improve the accuracy at
the boundaries. We conducted two experiments. To evaluate image synthesis, we investigated dependency of image synthesis accuracy on (1)
the number of training data and (2) incorporation of the gradient consistency loss. To demonstrate the applicability of our method, we also
investigated segmentation accuracy on synthesized images.

Keywords: Image synthesis · CycleGAN · Musculoskeletal image
MR · CT · Segmentation

1 Introduction

Computed tomography (CT) is commonly used in orthopedic procedures. Magnetic resonance imaging (MRI) is used along with CT to identify muscle structures and diagnose osteonecrosis due to its superior soft tissue contrast [1]. However, MRI has poor contrast for bone structures. It would be helpful if a corresponding CT were available, as bone boundaries are more clearly seen and CT

© Springer Nature Switzerland AG 2018
A. Gooya et al. (Eds.): SASHIMI 2018, LNCS 11037, pp. 31–41, 2018.
https://doi.org/10.1007/978-3-030-00536-8_4

has standardized (i.e., Hounsfield) units. Considering radiation exposure in CT, it is preferable if we can delineate boundaries of both muscle and bones in MRI. Therefore, we aim at MR-to-CT synthesis.

Image synthesis has been extensively studied using the patch-based learning [2] as well as deep learning, specifically, convolutional neural networks (CNN) [3] and generative adversarial networks (GAN) [4]. The conventional approaches required the paired training data, i.e., images of the same patient from multiple modalities that are registered, which limited the application. A method recently proposed by Zhu et al. [5], called CycleGAN, utilizes the unpaired training data by appreciating the cycle consistency loss function. While CycleGAN has already applied to MR-to-CT synthesis [6], all these previous approaches in medical image application targeted CT and MRI of the head in which the scan protocol (i.e., field-of-view (FOV) and the head orientation within the FOV) is relatively consistent resulting in a small variation in the two image distributions even without registration, thus a small number of training data set (20 to 30) allowed a reasonable accuracy. On the other hand, our target anatomy, the hip region, has larger variation in the anatomy as well as their pose (i.e., joint angle change and deformation of muscles).

Applications of image synthesis include segmentation. Some previous studies aimed at segmentation of musculoskeletal structures in MRI [7,8], but the issues in these studies were the requirement for multiple sequences and devices. Another challenge in segmentation of MRI is that there is no standard unit as in CT. Therefore, manually traced label data are necessary for training of each sequence and each imaging device. Thus, MR-to-CT synthesis realizes modality independent segmentation [9].

In this study, we extend the CycleGAN approach by adding the gradient consistency (GC) loss to encourage edge alignment between images in the two domains and using an order-of-magnitude larger training data set (302 MR and 613 CT volumes) in order to overcome the larger variation and improve the accuracy at the boundaries. We investigated dependency of image synthesis accuracy on 1) the number of training data and 2) incorporation of the GC loss. To demonstrate the applicability of our method, we also investigated a segmentation accuracy on synthesized images.

2 Method

2.1 Materials

The datasets we used in this study are MRI dataset consisting of 302 unlabeled volumes and CT dataset consisting of 613 unlabeled, and 20 labeled volumes which are associated with manual segmentation labels of 19 muscles around hip and thigh, pelvis, femur and sacrum bones. Patients with metallic artifact due to implant in the volume were excluded. As an evaluation dataset, we also used other three sets of paired MR and CT volumes, and 10 MR volumes associated with manual segmentation labels of gluteus medius and minimus muscles, pelvis and femur bones, as a ground truth. MR volumes were scanned in the coronal

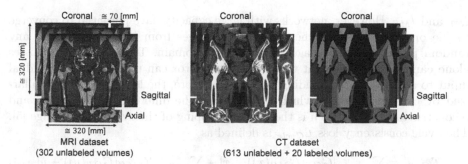

Fig. 1. Training datasets used in this study. MRI dataset consists of 302 unlabeled volumes and CT dataset consists of 613 unlabeled and 20 labeled volumes. N4ITK intensity inhomogeneity correction [10] was applied to all MRI volumes. Two datasets have similar field-of-view, although these are not registered.

plane for diagnosis of osteonecrosis by a 1.0T MR imaging system. The T1-weighted volumes were obtained by 3D spoiled gradient recalled echo sequence (SPGR) with a repetition time (TR) of 7.9 ms, echo time (TE) of 3.08 ms, and flip angle of 30. The field of view was 320 mm, and the matrix size was 256×256. The slab thickness was 76 mm, and the slice thickness was 2 mm without an inter-slice gap. CT volumes were scanned in the axial plane for diagnosis of the patients subjected to total hip arthroplasty (THA) surgery. The field of view was 360×360 mm and the matrix size was 512×512. The slice thickness was 2.0 mm for the region including pelvis and proximal femur, 6.0 mm for the femoral shaft region, and 1.0 mm for the distal femur region. In this study, the CT volumes were cropped and resliced so that the FOV resembles that of MRI volumes, as shown in Fig. 1, and then resized to 256×256.

2.2 Image Synthesis Using CycleGAN with Gradient-Consistency Loss

The underlying algorithm of the proposed MR-to-CT synthesis follows that of Zhu et al. [5] which allows to translate an image from CT domain to MR domain without pairwise aligned CT and MR training images of the same patient. The workflow of the proposed method is shown in Fig. 2. The networks G_{CT} and G_{MR} are generators to translate real MR and CT images to synthesized CT and MR images, respectivery. The networks D_{CT} and D_{MR} are discriminators to distinguish between real and synthesized images. While discriminators try to distinguish synthesized images by maximizing adversarial losses $\mathcal{L}_{CT}$ and $\mathcal{L}_{MR}$, defined as

$$\mathcal{L}_{CT} = \sum_{x \in I_{CT}} \log D_{CT}(x) + \sum_{y \in I_{MR}} \log(1 - D_{CT}(G_{CT}(y))), \quad (1)$$
$$\mathcal{L}_{MR} = \sum_{y \in I_{MR}} \log D_{MR}(y) + \sum_{x \in I_{CT}} \log(1 - D_{MR}(G_{MR}(x))), \quad (2)$$

generators try to synthesize images which is indistinguishable from the target domain by minimizing these losses. Where x and y are images from domains

I_{CT} and I_{MR}. However, networks with large capacity have potential to converge to the one that translate the same set of images from source domain to any random permutation of images in the target domain. Thus, adversarial losses alone cannot guarantee that the learned generator can translate an individual input to a desired corresponding output. Therefore, the loss function is regularized by cycle consistency, which is defined by the difference between real and reconstructed image, which is the inverse mapping of the synthesized image [5]. The cycle consistency loss $\mathcal{L}_{Cycle}$ is defined as

$$\mathcal{L}_{Cycle} = \sum_{x \in I_{CT}} |G_{CT}(G_{MR}(x)) - x| + \sum_{y \in I_{MR}} |G_{MR}(G_{CT}(y)) - y| \quad (3)$$

We extended the CycleGAN approach by explicitly adding the gradient consistency loss between real and synthesized images to improve the accuracy at the boundaries. The gradient correlation (GC) [11] has been used as a similarity metric in the medical image registration, which is defined by the normalized cross correlation between two images. Given gradients in horizontal and vertical directions of these two images, A and B, GC is defined as

$$GC(A, B) = \frac{1}{2}\{NCC(\nabla_x A, \nabla_x B) + NCC(\nabla_y A, \nabla_y B)\} \quad (4)$$

$$\text{where,} \quad NCC(A, B) = \frac{\sum_{(i,j)}(A - \bar{A})(B - \bar{B})}{\sqrt{\sum_{(i,j)}(A - \bar{A})^2}\sqrt{\sum_{(i,j)}(B - \bar{B})^2}}$$

and ∇_x and ∇_y are the gradient operator of each direction, $\bar{A}$ is the mean value of A. We formulate the gradient-consistency loss $\mathcal{L}_{GC}$ as

$$\mathcal{L}_{GC} = \frac{1}{2}\{\sum_{x \in I_{CT}} (1 - GC(x, G_{MR}(x))) + \sum_{y \in I_{MR}} (1 - GC(y, G_{CT}(y)))\} \quad (5)$$

Finally, our objective function is defined as:

$$\mathcal{L}_{total} = \mathcal{L}_{CT} + \mathcal{L}_{MR} + \lambda_{Cycle}\mathcal{L}_{Cycle} + \lambda_{GC}\mathcal{L}_{GC} \quad (6)$$

where λ_{Cycle} and λ_{GC} are weights to balance each loss. Then, we solve:

$$\hat{G}_{MR}, \hat{G}_{CT} = \arg \min_{G_{CT}, G_{MR}} \max_{D_{CT}, D_{MR}} \mathcal{L}_{total} \quad (7)$$

In this paper, we used 2D CNN with 9 residual blocks for generator, similar to the one proposed in [12]. For discriminators, we used 70×70 PatchGAN [13]. We replaced the Eqs. (1) and (2) by least-squares loss as in [14]. These settings follows [5,6]. The CycleGAN was trained using Adam [15] for the first 1×10^5 iterations at fixed learning rate of 0.0002, and the last 1×10^5 iterations at learning rate which linearly reducing to zero. The balancing weights were empirically determined as $\lambda_{Cycle} = 3$ and $\lambda_{GC} = 0.3$. CT and MR volumes are normalized such that intensity of $[-150, 350]$ HU and $[0, 100]$ are mapped to $[0, 255]$, respectively.

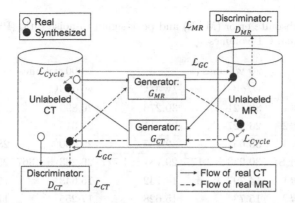

Fig. 2. Workflow of the proposed method. G_{CT} and G_{MR} are generator networks that translate MR to CT images, and CT to MR images, respectively. D_{CT} and D_{MR} are discriminator networks to distinguish between real and synthesized images. The cycle consistency loss $\mathcal{L}_{Cycle}$ is a regularization term defined by the difference between real and reconstructed image. To improve the accuracy at the edges, loss function is regularized by gradient consistency loss $\mathcal{L}_{GC}$.

3   Result

3.1   Quantitative Evaluation on Image Synthesis

To evaluate image synthesis, we investigated dependency of the accuracy on the number of training data and with or without the GC loss. The CycleGAN was trained with datasets of different sizes, (i) 20 MR and 20 CT volumes, (ii) 302 MR and 613 CT volumes, and both with and without GC loss. We conducted two experiments. The first experiment used three sets of paired MR and CT volumes of the same patient for test data. Because availability of paired MR and CT volumes was limited, we conducted the second experiment in which unpaired 10 MR and 20 CT volumes were used.

In the first experiment, we evaluated synthesized CT by means of mean absolute error (MAE) and peak-signal-to-noise ratio (PSNR) [dB] between synthesized CT and ground truth CT, both of which were normalized as mentioned in 2.2. The ground truth CT here is a CT registered to the MR of the same patient. CT and MR volumes were aligned using landmark-based registration as initialization, and then aligned using rigid and non-rigid registration. The results of MAE and PSNR are shown in Table 1. PSNR is calculated as $PSNR = 20 \log_{10} \frac{255}{\sqrt{MSE}}$, where MSE is mean squared error. The average of MAE decreased and PSNR increased according to the increase of training data size and inclusion of GC loss, respectively. Figure 3 shows representative results.

In the second experiment, we tested with unpaired 10 MR and 20 CT volumes. Mutual information (MI) between synthesized CT and original MR was used for evaluation when the paired ground truth was not available. The quantitative results are show in Fig. 4(a). The left side is the box and whisker plots

Table 1. Mean absolute error (MAE) and peak-signal-to-noise ratio (PSNR) between synthesized and real CT volumes.

		20 volumes		>300 volumes	
		w/o GC	/w GC	w/o GC	/w GC
MAE	Patient #1	30.121	30.276	26.899	26.388
	Patient #2	26.927	26.911	22.319	21.593
	Patient #3	33.651	32.155	29.630	28.643
	Average ± SD	30.233 ± 2.177	29.781 ± 1.777	26.283 ± 1.367	25.541 ± 1.129
PSNR	Patient #1	14.797	14.742	15.643	15.848
	Patient #2	15.734	15.628	17.255	17.598
	Patient #3	14.510	14.820	15.674	15.950
	Average ± SD	15.014 ± 0.330	15.063 ± 0.380	16.190 ± 0.273	16.465 ± 0.296

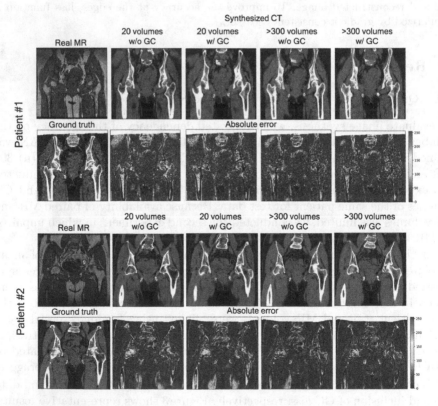

Fig. 3. Representative results of the absolute error between the ground truth paired CT and synthesized CT from two patients. Since the FOV of MR and CT volumes are slightly different, there is no corresponding region near the top edge of the ground truth volumes (filled with white color). This area was not used for evaluation.

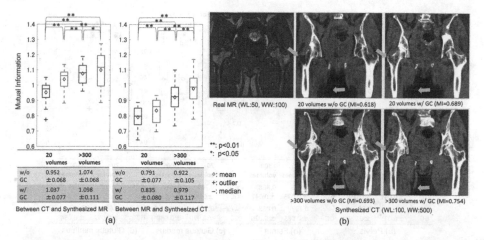

	20 volumes	>300 volumes		20 volumes	>300 volumes
w/o GC	0.952 ±0.068	1.074 ±0.068	w/o GC	0.791 ±0.077	0.922 ±0.105
w/ GC	1.037 ±0.077	1.098 ±0.111	w/ GC	0.835 ±0.080	0.979 ±0.117

Between CT and Synthesized MR   Between MR and Synthesized CT

**: p<0.01
*: p<0.05

◇: mean
+: outlier
−: median

(a)

(b)

Fig. 4. Evaluation of similarity between the real and synthesized volumes. (a) quantitative comparison of mutual information on different training data size with and without the gradient-consistency loss. (b) representative result of one patient.

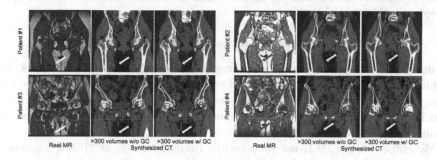

Fig. 5. Representative results of translation from real MR to synthesized CT of four patients with and without the gradient consistency loss. As indicated by arrows, synthesized volumes with gradient consistency loss helped to preserve the shape near the adductor muscles.

of the mean of each slice of MI between real CT and synthesized MR (i.e., 20 data points in total). The right side is the mean of MI between real MR and synthesized CT (i.e., 10 data points in total). The result shows that the larger number of training data yielded statistically significant improvement ($p < 0.01$) according to the paired t-test in MI. The GC loss also leads to an increase in MI between MR and synthesized CT ($p < 0.01$). Figures 4(b) and 5 show examples of the visualization of real MR and synthesized CT volumes. As indicated by arrows, we can see that synthesized volumes with GC loss preserved the shape near the femoral head and adductor muscles.

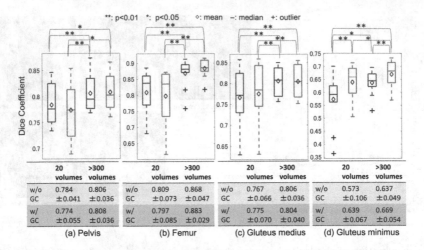

Fig. 6. Evaluation of segmentation accuracy on different training data size in Cycle-GAN with and without the gradient-consistency loss. Segmentation of (a) pelvis, (b) femur, (c) gluteus medius and (d) gluteus minimus muscle in MR volumes were performed using MR-to-CT synthesis.

3.2 Quantitative Evaluation on Segmentation

To demonstrate the applicability of image synthesis in segmentation task, we evaluated the segmentation accuracy. Twenty labeled CT datasets were used to train the segmentation network. Then, we evaluated the segmentation accuracy with 10 MR volumes with manual segmentation labels of the gluteus medius and minimus muscles and femur.

We employed the 2D U-net proposed by Ronneberger et al. [16] as segmentation network, which is widely used in medical image analysis and demonstrated high performance with a limited number of labeled volumes. In MRI, muscle boundaries are clearer while bone boundaries are clearer in CT. To incorporate the advantage of both CT and MR, we modified the 2D U-net to take the two-channel input of both CT and synthesized MR images. We trained on 2D U-net using Adam [15] for 1×10^5 iterations at learning rate of 0.0001. At the test phase, a pair of MR and synthesized CT was used as two-channel input.

The results with 4 musculoskeletal structures for 10 patients are shown in Fig. 6 (i.e., 10 data points in total on each plot). The result shows that the larger number of training data yielded statistically significant improvement in DICE on pelvis ($p < 0.01$), femur ($p < 0.01$), glutes medius ($p < 0.01$) and glutes minimus regions ($p < 0.05$) of paired t-test. The GC loss also leads to an increase in DICE on the glutes minimus regions ($p < 0.01$). The average DICE coefficient in the cases trained with more than 300 cases and GC loss was 0.808 ± 0.036 (pelvis), 0.883 ± 0.029 (femur), 0.804 ± 0.040 (gluteus medius) and 0.669 ± 0.054 (gluteus minimus), respectively. Figure 7 shows example visualization of real MR, synthesized CT, and estimated label for one patient. The result with GC loss has smoother segmentation not only in the gluteus minimus but also near the adductor muscles.

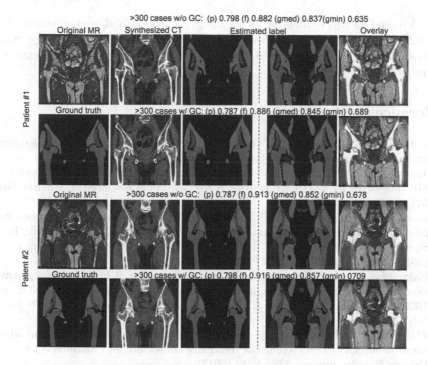

Fig. 7. Representative results of segmentation from one patient. The ground truth label is consist of 4 musculoskeletal structures in MRI. Although we evaluated only on 4 structures because ground truth were not available for the other structures on MRI, all 22 estimated labels are shown for qualitative evaluation. In the right-most column, all estimated labels are overlayed on the real MRI. p, f, gmed, gmin denote DICE of pelvis, femur, gluteus medius, and gluteus minimus, respectively.

4   Discussion and Conclusion

In this study, we proposed an image synthesis method which extended the Cycle-GAN approach by adding the GC loss to improve the accuracy at the boundaries. Specifically, the contributions of this paper are (1) introduction of GC loss in CycleGAN, and (2) quantitative and qualitative evaluation of the dependency of both image synthesis accuracy and segmentation accuracy on a large number of training data. One limitation in this study is that we excluded the patients with implants, while our target cohort (i.e., THA patients) sometime has implant on one side, for example, in case of the planning of secondary surgery. As a comparison against a single modality training, we performed 5-fold cross validation of MR segmentation using 10 labeled MR volumes (i.e., trained with 8 MR volumes and tested on remaining 2 MR volumes) using U-net segmentation network. The DICE was 0.815 ± 0.046 (pelvis), 0.921 ± 0.023 (femur), 0.825 ± 0.029 (gluteus medius) and 0.752 ± 0.045 (gluteus minimus), respectively. We found the gap of accuracy between modality independent and dependent segmentation. A potential improvement of modality independent segmentation is to construct an end-to-end network that performs image synthesis and segmentation [17]. Our future work also includes development of a method that effectively incorporates information in unlabeled CT and MR volumes to improve segmentation accuracy [18].

References

1. Cvitanic, O.: MRI diagnosis of tears of the hip abductor tendons (gluteus medius and gluteus minimus). Am. J. Roentgenol. **182**(1), 137–143 (2004)
2. Torrado-Carvajal, A.: Fast patch-based pseudo-CT synthesis from T1-weighted MR images for PET/MR attenuation correction in brain studies. J. Nuclear Med. **57**(1), 136–143 (2016)
3. Zhao, C., Carass, A., Lee, J., He, Y., Prince, J.L.: Whole brain segmentation and labeling from CT using synthetic MR images. In: Wang, Q., Shi, Y., Suk, H.-I., Suzuki, K. (eds.) MLMI 2017. LNCS, vol. 10541, pp. 291–298. Springer, Cham (2017). https://doi.org/10.1007/978-3-319-67389-9_34
4. Kamnitsas, K., et al.: Unsupervised domain adaptation in brain lesion segmentation with adversarial networks. In: Niethammer, M. (ed.) IPMI 2017. LNCS, vol. 10265, pp. 597–609. Springer, Cham (2017). https://doi.org/10.1007/978-3-319-59050-9_47
5. Zhu, J.Y., et al.: Unpaired image-to-image translation using cycle-consistent adversarial networks. In: Proceedings of the IEEE Conference on Computer Vision and Pattern Recognition, pp. 2223–2232 (2017)
6. Wolterink, J.M., Dinkla, A.M., Savenije, M.H.F., Seevinck, P.R., van den Berg, C.A.T., Išgum, I.: Deep MR to CT synthesis using unpaired data. In: Tsaftaris, S.A., Gooya, A., Frangi, A.F., Prince, J.L. (eds.) SASHIMI 2017. LNCS, vol. 10557, pp. 14–23. Springer, Cham (2017). https://doi.org/10.1007/978-3-319-68127-6_2
7. Gilles, B.: Musculoskeletal MRI segmentation using multi-resolution simplex meshes with medial representations. Med. Image Anal. **14**(3), 291–302 (2010)
8. Ranzini, M.B.M., et al.: Joint multimodal segmentation of clinical CT and MR from hip arthroplasty patients. In: Glocker, B., Yao, J., Vrtovec, T., Frangi, A., Zheng, G. (eds.) MSKI 2017. LNCS, vol. 10734, pp. 72–84. Springer, Cham (2018). https://doi.org/10.1007/978-3-319-74113-0_7
9. Hamarneh, G., Jassi, P., Tang, L.: Simulation of ground-truth validation data via physically-and statistically-based warps. In: Metaxas, D., Axel, L., Fichtinger, G., Székely, G. (eds.) MICCAI 2008. LNCS, vol. 5241, pp. 459–467. Springer, Heidelberg (2008). https://doi.org/10.1007/978-3-540-85988-8_55
10. Tustison, N.J.: N4ITK: improved N3 bias correction. IEEE Trans. Med. Imaging **29**(6), 1310–1320 (2010)
11. Penney, G.P.: A comparison of similarity measures for use in 2-D-3-D medical image registration. IEEE Trans. Med. Imaging **17**(4), 586–595 (1998)
12. Johnson, J., Alahi, A., Fei-Fei, L.: Perceptual losses for real-time style transfer and super-resolution. In: Leibe, B., Matas, J., Sebe, N., Welling, M. (eds.) ECCV 2016. LNCS, vol. 9906, pp. 694–711. Springer, Cham (2016). https://doi.org/10.1007/978-3-319-46475-6_43
13. Isola, P., et al.: Image-to-image translation with conditional adversarial networks. arXiv preprint (2017)
14. Mao, X., et al.: Multi-class generative adversarial networks with the L2 loss function. CoRR, abs/1611.04076 2 (2016)

15. Kingma, D.P., et al.: Adam: a method for stochastic optimization. arXiv preprint arXiv:1412.6980 (2014)
16. Ronneberger, O., Fischer, P., Brox, T.: U-Net: convolutional networks for biomedical image segmentation. In: Navab, N., Hornegger, J., Wells, W.M., Frangi, A.F. (eds.) MICCAI 2015. LNCS, vol. 9351, pp. 234–241. Springer, Cham (2015). https://doi.org/10.1007/978-3-319-24574-4_28
17. Huo, Y., et al.: Adversarial synthesis learning enables segmentation without target modality ground truth. arXiv preprint arXiv:1712.07695 (2017)
18. Zhang, Y., Yang, L., Chen, J., Fredericksen, M., Hughes, D.P., Chen, D.Z.: Deep adversarial networks for biomedical image segmentation utilizing unannotated images. In: Descoteaux, M., Maier-Hein, L., Franz, A., Jannin, P., Collins, D.L., Duchesne, S. (eds.) MICCAI 2017. LNCS, vol. 10435, pp. 408–416. Springer, Cham (2017). https://doi.org/10.1007/978-3-319-66179-7_47

A Machine Learning Approach to Diffusion MRI Partial Volume Estimation

Emmanuel Vallee[1(✉)], Wenchuan Wu[1], Francesca Galassi[2], Saad Jbabdi[1],
and Stephen Smith[1]

[1] FMRIB Analysis Group, NDCN, University of Oxford, Oxford, UK
`manu.vallee@gmail.com`
[2] INRIA, CNRS UMR6074, VISAGES: INSERM U1228, University of Rennes I,
Rennes, France

Abstract. Tissue-type partial volume modelling is generally an ill-posed problem in single-shell diffusion MRI. On the other hand, T1w images are typically acquired along with the diffusion data, and allow for an accurate estimation of the tissue partial volume fractions (PVFs). We propose in this paper to compare different data driven approach to predict the T1w-derived PVFs from the diffusion data. The aim is to alleviate the within subject mis-registration between the two modalities.

Our experiments show that the random forests is the most accurate and scalable method for predicting the tissue partial volume fractions. Additionally, such predictions can be used to inform the fitting of the two-compartment model to retrieve a diffusion tensor that is not biased by partial volume effects or constraints.

Keywords: Diffusion MRI · Multi-compartment models
Machine learning

1 Introduction

The presence of free water (FW) in a white matter (WM) voxel is known to confound the interpretation of the diffusion tensor indices [10]. However, fitting a multi-compartment diffusion MRI model that includes a FW compartment is an ill-posed problem, as it often requires spatial regularisation or the introduction of prior knowledge for the tissue compartment [12,14]. These regularisation schemes potentially reduce the sensitivity of the tensor indices to WM alteration (e.g., in pathology). Additionally, the voxel-wise fitting of the FW model estimates a non-zero CSF volume fraction in deep WM, where it is expected to be zero [13].

A T1w image is usually acquired along with the diffusion sequence in a typical study. T1w images generally have high resolution, good SNR and a high contrast between tissues. We propose here to use the CSF PVF estimated from the T1w image as a prior in order to fit a two-compartment model on the diffusion data.

© Springer Nature Switzerland AG 2018
A. Gooya et al. (Eds.): SASHIMI 2018, LNCS 11037, pp. 42–51, 2018.
https://doi.org/10.1007/978-3-030-00536-8_5

We hypothesize that the extra information can improve the stability of the fitting and allow to relax the constraint on the MD.

A similar approach was previously proposed in [5]. However, the crucial issue of mis-registration between the T1w image and the diffusion data was not addressed. In a typical study, susceptibility-induced distortions associated with the echo planar imaging (EPI) and the eddy current induced distortions limit the accuracy of the co-registration. Susceptibility-induced distortions can be adressed using a separately acquired fieldmap that allows to accurately unwarp the EPI images [9]. Alternative methods can be used to estimate such fieldmap when the latter was not acquired in the experiment, but they require the acquisition of images with opposite phase-ecoding directions [2]. However, in many dMRI group studies, no fieldmap or opposite phase encoded images are available. Consequently, using directly co-registered T1w-derived tissue PVFs in a diffusion model may result in significant deviations in the estimation of the tensor FA or MD.

In order to avoid the co-registration issue, we propose to use a data-driven approach to learn a mapping between diffusion features and the tissues' PVFs estimated from the T1w images. Supervised machine learning methods have already been successfully applied in diffusion MRI. For example, it was shown that the NODDI model can be successfully fitted on single shell data by applying a random forest regression method [1].

In this work, we compare four supervised machine learning approaches in their ability to predict the tissue PVFs. We use a range of diffusion features estimated from models applicable to low b-value single-shell data, that is typically encountered in group studies. We also evaluate the robustness of our approach to the error in registration between the T1w and diffusion images. Finally, we use the CSF PVF predicted by our method as a prior while fitting the FW model and assess how the additional information relaxes the constraints on the diffusion tensor parameters.

2   Materials and Methods

2.1   Data Acquisition and Pre-processing

We performed our experiments on two similar datasets of two separate subjects. Data was acquired on a 3T Siemens Verio scanner. Diffusion data consisted of a standard DWI acquisition with $TR = 9600$ ms, $TE = 76$ ms and $b = 1000 \, s \, mm^{-2}$, with 60 non-collinear diffusion gradient directions in addition to 6 non-weighted $b = 0$ images. The voxel size was 2 mm isotropic, with a parallel imaging acceleration factor of 2, for a total scan time of 12 min. The structural $T1w$ image was acquired at a resolution of 1 mm isotropic for a scan time of 6 min.

Another set of diffusion data was also acquired, consisting of an Inversion Recovery (IR) sequence where the CSF signal was nulled. The acquisition parameters were: $TR = 20.6$ s, $TI = 2300$ ms, $b = 1000 \, s \, mm^{-2}$, with 60 non-collinear diffusion gradient directions in addition to 6 non-weighted $b = 0$ images. This acquisition allows retrieving tensor indices that are not contaminated by the CSF contribution to the signal [11].

The diffusion data was preprocessed to correct for movement and eddy currents distortions with EDDY [3]. The diffusion features consisted of 17 parameters resulting from: the DWIs (mean b0, mean b1000), the diffusion tensor (FA, MD, tensor mode and the 3 tensor eigenvalues), Ball&Stick model [4] (volume fractions of the 3 fibres, total fibre volume fraction, isotropic diffusivity and the dispersion of the 3 fibres orientations) and finally probabilistic tractography (visitation maps for full brain tractography). In order to add information from the neighbouring voxels, we added a smoothed version of each feature map ($\sigma =$ 6 mm) as well as its gradient, for a total of 51 features.

The tissue PVFs were estimated on the T1w image using FAST [17]. These PVFs were then registered to the diffusion data with FLIRT BBR [7].

2.2   Predicting Tissues Volume Fraction

Our method relies on a voxel-wise regression, that learns a mapping between the features derived from the diffusion data and the corresponding tissue PVFs computed on the T1w image. A supervised machine learning (ML) approach requires a training and a testing dataset. In our case, training is performed on one subject and testing on another subject. To train the ML model, we assume that T1 and diffusion images are accurately registered.

2.3   Comparison of the Machine Learning Approaches

We compare the performance of 4 machine learning approaches: random forest (RF), support vector machine regression (SVR), Gaussian process (GP) and neural networks (NN). The methods' hyper-parameters were optimised using grid search for the RF and SVR, gradient descent for the Gaussian process and an empirical manner for the NN. The optimisation of the 4 ML approaches (RF, SVR, GP and NN) was based on the correlation between the predictions and the T1 segmentation on a validation set, except for the GP, where the parameters were optimised only on the training set. Each of the 4 methods was optimised on the same set of 20000 voxels.

The performance of each ML approach was similarly assessed with the correlation between their PVF predictions and the PVF estimated from the T1, for each tissue (WM, GM and CSF). The correlation was computed on the full brain of the test subject. It ensured that the performance measure includes false positives, e.g. non-zero WM volume fraction in the CSF as well as false negatives, e.g. zero WM volume fraction in the middle of the white matter.

2.4   Mis-registration Between T1 and Diffusion Space

The main motivations to use a ML approach is the mis-registration between T1 and diffusion space. Therefore, we evaluated how the registration error affects the performance of the learning process. We introduced additional registration error between structural and diffusion data on the learning dataset, and computed how the performance of the segmentation on the test dataset was impacted.

2.5 Application to FW Modelling

In this experiment, we fitted the FW model described in [14]. We used the predicted CSF volume fraction as a prior for the FW compartment. The mean of the prior is equal to the volume fraction predicted, with a correction factor to account for the different T1 and T2 relaxation times of the tissues, with $FWF = \frac{\hat{S}_{fw}}{\hat{S}_{fw} + \hat{S}_T}$, where $S_X = \hat{S}_X(1 - \exp[-TR/T_{1,X}]) \exp[-TE/T_{2,X}]$. The standard deviation of the tissue PVF prior is set to 0.1, which approximately corresponds to the standard deviation of the error between our model prediction and the T1 segmentation. Compared to [14], we relaxed the prior on the MD, with its standard deviation to $0.5 \times 10^{-3} \, \text{mm}^2 \, \text{s}^{-1}$.

3 Results

3.1 Machine Learning Approaches Comparison

The random forest optimal architecture consisted in 100 fully grown trees with 90% of the features used at each split. The SVR was an ϵ-SVR ($\epsilon - 0.01$) with a Gaussian kernel ($\gamma = 0.1$) and a regularisation parameter $C = 1$. The best perfomance for the Gaussian process was obtained with a Gaussian kernel with a length-scale of 3.6 and a noise level parameter of 0.1. Finally, the best NN architecture consisted in 3 hidden layers with 200 units each and a rectified linear activation function.

In Fig. 1, we show the performance obtained with the 4 ML approaches for the 3 tissue types. Overall, the RF exhibits the highest correlation between the predictions and the T1 segmentation, for the 3 tissue types ($r = 0.83$, 0.88 and 0.93 for the CSF, GM and WM respectively). It is closely followed by the NN. The SVR and GP perform less well. In addition to its high accuracy, the random forest method was also the fastest. The training phase was performed in a few minutes, whereas the other methods required a few hours.

Figure 2 shows the segmentation maps predicted by the RF method, as well as the T1w image segmentation. For a given voxel, the tissue with the highest PVF is represented. Visually, the RF segmentation maps are very similar to the T1 segmentation. The RF still gives high WM PVF prediction in the crossing areas (>0.95). We note that the RF segmentation is better in the subcortical structures as they contains higher GM PVFs.

3.2 Mis-registration Between T1 and Diffusion Space

Figure 3 shows the correlation and MSE obtained on the test dataset as a function of the mis-registration (translation along the x, y and z axes) artificially

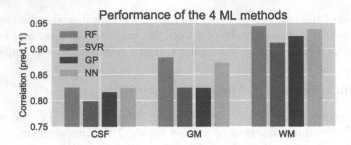

Fig. 1. Comparison of the four ML approaches. Correlation between T1w-derived and predicted (from diffusion data) partial volume segmentation using random forest (RF), Gaussian process (GP) and support vector regression (SVR).

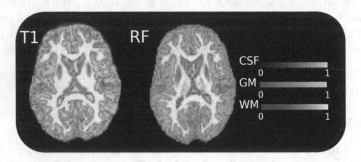

Fig. 2. Segmentation maps predicted with the RF method. Tissues' partial volume fraction obtained from the T1 and RF method in diffusion space.

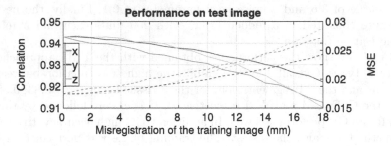

Fig. 3. Impact of the mis-registration on the RF performance. Correlation and MSE between predicted and ground truth PVF on the test data as a function of the misregistration between diffusion and structural space on the training data.

introduced into the training dataset. To compute the scores, we used the RF regression. The plots show that the correlation is at its maximum when there is no mis-registration, reaching 0.943, with an MSE of 0.017. The correlation gradually decreases (and the MSE increases) as the registration error increases. Interestingly, we see that a mis-registration along the x axis (left-right orientation) has more impact on the performance than in the y and z axes.

Here, the key result is that the method is very robust to misregistration of the training dataset. Indeed, the correlation and the MSE obtained on the test dataset stays almost constant when the training error remains under 2 mm, which corresponds to the voxel size of our diffusion data. The robustness of our approach validates its applicability to datasets where EPI distortions are significant and cannot be corrected.

3.3 Synthetic T1

We performed an additional experiment to predict the absolute T1 intensities at their native resolution (1 mm), using RF and the diffusion features up-sampled to 1mm. In the Fig. 4, the RF predictions are shown together with the T1w original image in the same space. We observe that the predictions look very similar to the original T1w image, and the correlation coefficient between the two images is high ($r = 0.948$). The contrast between grey and white matter is excellent on the original T1w image, as expected from this modality. The WM/GM contrast is also very good in the predictions. This is an interesting result, given that the prediction is obtained from a single-shell acquisition.

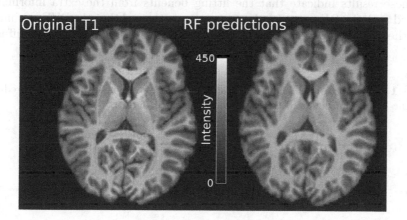

Fig. 4. Prediction of T1w image intensities. Original T1w and T1w image predicted with the random forest from upsampled diffusion data

The main outcome of this experiment is the quality of the predictions in terms of resolution. Although the diffusion features were derived from data with a resolution of 2 mm, the predictions at 1 mm appear excellent. The predicted T1w is slightly blurrier than the original one, but the actual resolution is very close to the original T1w. In term of the resolution element (RESEL) [15] the original T1w linear RESEL is 17.2 mm and the predicted T1w RESEL is 19.4 mm. The latter is lower than the RESEL obtained with spline interpolation, which is in this case 22.5 mm. Importantly, this result shows that our method takes advantage of the sub-voxel "super-resolution" information contained in the diffusion data.

3.4 Application to FW Modelling

We show here how the prior (derived from the RF predictions) on the CSF compartment affects the fitting of the FW model to the diffusion data. We used the RF predictions, as they are the most accurate. As a reference, we also included the results obtained with the T1-derived CSF PVFs, which are prone to registration error. Finally, we show the results obtained with the same model, without the prior on the CSF volume fraction.

In Table 1, we show the FA and MD obtained in the regions where partial voluming between the CSF and the WM occurs. These regions are defined by a WM PVF ≥ 0.5, a CSF PVF ≥ 0.1, and a GM PVF $= 0$. We compare our fitting with the inversion recovery acquisition where the CSF signal was nulled. We indicated the correlation as well as the MSE, the latter being more sensitive to biased estimates. The table shows that the best results (in bold) are obtained when we used the CSF PVFs predicted by the random forest as a prior on the FW volume fraction. Importantly, when we used the RF CSF prior, the CSF PVF estimated in the deep WM was constant with a value of 0. When the prior is not used, the model estimates a non-zero FWF (on average 0.1) in crossing fibres areas, which affects the tissue MD and FA.

These results indicate that the fitting benefits from the extra information inferred with the RF approach. Importantly, we showed that the PVFs estimated from the T1 should not be directly used when fitting the model on the diffusion data.

Table 1. Correlation coefficient (r) and RMSE between the FA and MD predicted with the different priors and the inversion recovery ground truth.

Method	r (FA)	RMSE (FA)	r (MD)	RMSE (MD in $mm^2 s^{-1}$)
RF prior	**0.66**	**0.15**	**0.51**	**0.27**
T1 prior	0.57	0.19	0.35	0.31
no prior	0.62	0.17	0.49	0.34

4   Discussion

Machine Learning Approaches. Amongst the 4 machine learning techniques we evaluated, we found that the random forests outperforms other approaches. It is closely followed by the NN method, while the SVR and GP are both under-performing. This result is not unexpected, as the RF approach is known to be very efficient, scalable, and effective for a wide range of supervised learning problems. The neural network approach has been shown to be promising as well, although it requires a more careful tuning and is more computationally demanding than the RF. Additionally, the NN can be naturally extended to use the spatial neighbourhood with convolutional neural networks (CNN). We tried to use a 3D CNN method that was but we unfortunately faced implementation issues, as the optimisation of the weights in the context of regression proved to be difficult.

Diffusion Features. In this work, we employed diffusion features derived from well known models (diffusion tensor and ball and stick), as well as the tractography visitation map. One of the motivations was to make the method applicable to acquisitions with different parameters (e.g. number and orientation of diffusion gradients, resolution, number of b-values). Another motivation was that the features are rotationally independent, and therefore they do not require the training and testing datasets to be aligned. A model free approach was used in [6]. The signal intensities from each diffusion gradient were directly used as features in order to infer NODDI and DKI parameters. While their approach appears to be promising, it is restricted to the case where the same diffusion protocol is used for an entire study.

Diffusion Data Segmentation. We successfully applied our ML approaches to partial volume segmentation. The segmentation maps appeared homogeneous, even though no spatial regularisation was used. However, it heavily relies on the accuracy of the T1 segmentation, which was inaccurate, notably in the sub-cortical grey matter structures. FAST, being purely driven by the voxelwise T1w intensities, generally does not give good thalamus segmentation, whereas the dMRI-based PVF prediction more accurately estimated larger GM content in the thalamus.

Application to FW Modelling. The first motivation of our work was to improve the fitting of a two-compartment model that accounts for CSF contamination. By adding an informative prior on the CSF volume fraction, we were able to prevent the model from fitting a CSF compartment in deep white matter. As a result, the micro-structural properties estimated in the tissue are not biased either by the MD prior or by the presence of a spurious CSF compartment. Secondly, the CSF PVF prior enables us to relax the prior on the MD. We showed that the extra information provided by the RF reduces the bias on the MD estimated by the model in areas where partial volume effects are present. We note that our work could easily be extended to a more complex diffusion model with a CSF compartment, such as NODDI [16], or models with a GM compartment, such as multi-tissue spherical deconvolution [8].

Implications for the Future. The analysis of diffusion data was until recently exclusively based on an explicit model that often require advanced diffusion acquisition protocols. Our results showed that a machine learning approach can provide extra-information that is useful for solving ill-posed problems. A corollary is that the diffusion data contains redundant information. It was indeed demonstrated that a machine learning approach (neural networks) can reduce the amount of data needed to fit NODDI model by a factor of 12 [6]. In another study, it was shown that using an ML based approach can infer NODDI microstructural parameters more accurately than a direct fitting on the data [13]. They showed that their method is robust to mesoscopic changes of the white matter (i.e., the geometric padding of the fibres).

5   Conclusion

In this work, we showed the potential of ML approaches to retrieve quantities from the diffusion data that cannot be derived with an explicit model. Our experiments were limited to one test subject, as inversion recovery DWI data is uncommon in larger dataset. Finally, on top of ensuring anatomical accuracy, our method also provides useful information that allows to retrieve unbiased tensor indices throughout the entire WM.

References

1. Alexander, D.C., et al.: Image quality transfer and applications in diffusion MRI. NeuroImage 152, 283–298 (2017)
2. Andersson, J.L.R., Skare, S., Ashburner, J.: How to correct susceptibility distortions in spin-echo echo-planar images: application to diffusion tensor imaging. NeuroImage 20(2), 870–888 (2003)
3. Andersson, J.L., Sotiropoulos, S.N.: An integrated approach to correction for off-resonance effects and subject movement in diffusion MR imaging. Neuroimage 125, 1063–1078 (2016)
4. Behrens, T.E.J., Berg, H.J., Jbabdi, S., Rushworth, M.F.S., Woolrich, M.W.: Probabilistic diffusion tractography with multiple fibre orientations: what can we gain? NeuroImage 34(1), 144–155 (2007)
5. Eaton-Rosen, Z., Melbourne, A., Cardoso, M.J., Marlow, N., Ourselin, S.: Beyond the resolution limit: diffusion parameter estimation in partial volume. In: Ourselin, S., Joskowicz, L., Sabuncu, M.R., Unal, G., Wells, W. (eds.) MICCAI 2016. LNCS, vol. 9902, pp. 605–612. Springer, Cham (2016). https://doi.org/10.1007/978-3-319-46726-9_70
6. Golkov, V.: q-Space deep learning: twelve-fold shorter and model-free diffusion MRI scans. IEEE Trans. Med. Imaging 35(5), 1344–1351 (2016)
7. Greve, D.N., Fischl, B.: Accurate and robust brain image alignment using boundary-based registration. NeuroImage 48(1), 63–72 (2009)
8. Jeurissen, B., Tournier, J.D., Dhollander, T., Connelly, A., Sijbers, J.: Multi-tissue constrained spherical deconvolution for improved analysis of multi-shell diffusion MRI data. NeuroImage 103, 411–426 (2014)
9. Jezzard, P., Balaban, R.S.: Correction for geometric distortion in echo planar images from B0 field variations. Magn. Reson. Med. 34(1), 65–73 (1995)
10. Metzler-Baddeley, C., O'Sullivan, M.J., Bells, S., Pasternak, O., Jones, D.K.: How and how not to correct for CSF-contamination in diffusion MRI. NeuroImage 59(2), 1394–1403 (2012)

11. Papadakis, N.G., et al.: Study of the effect of CSF suppression on white matter diffusion anisotropy mapping of healthy human brain. Magn. Reson. Med. **48**(2), 394–398 (2002)
12. Pasternak, O., Sochen, N., Gur, Y., Intrator, N., Assaf, Y.: Free water elimination and mapping from diffusion MRI. Magn. Reson. Med. **62**(3), 717–730 (2009)
13. Reisert, M., Kellner, E., Dhital, B., Hennig, J., Kiselev, V.G.: Disentangling micro from mesostructure by diffusion MRI: a Bayesian approach. NeuroImage **147**, 964–975 (2017)
14. Vallee, E., et al.: Modelling free water in diffusion MRI. In: Proceedings of the International Society for Magnetic Resonance in Medicine, Abstract 0474 (2015)
15. Worsley, K.J., Evans, A.C., Marrett, S., Neelin, P.: A three-dimensional statistical analysis for CBF activation studies in human brain. J. Cereb. Blood Flow Metab. **12**(6), 900–918 (1992)
16. Zhang, H., Schneider, T., Wheeler-Kingshott, C.A., Alexander, D.C.: NODDI: practical in vivo neurite orientation dispersion and density imaging of the human brain. NeuroImage **61**(4), 1000–1016 (2012)
17. Zhang, Y., Brady, M., Smith, S.: Segmentation of brain MR images through a hidden Markov random field model and the expectation-maximization algorithm. IEEE Trans. Med. Imaging **20**(1), 45–57 (2001)

Unsupervised Learning for Cross-Domain Medical Image Synthesis Using Deformation Invariant Cycle Consistency Networks

Chengjia Wang[1,2]([✉]), Gillian Macnaught[1,2], Giorgos Papanastasiou[2],
Tom MacGillivray[2], and David Newby[1,2]

[1] BHF Centre for Cadiovascular Science, University of Edinburgh, Edinburgh, UK
chengjia.wang@ed.ac.uk
[2] Edinburgh Imaging Facility QMRI, University of Edinburgh, Edinburgh, UK

Abstract. Recently, the cycle-consistent generative adversarial networks (CycleGAN) has been widely used for synthesis of multi-domain medical images. The domain-specific nonlinear deformations captured by CycleGAN make the synthesized images difficult to be used for some applications, for example, generating pseudo-CT for PET-MR attenuation correction. This paper presents a deformation-invariant CycleGAN (DicycleGAN) method using deformable convolutional layers and new cycle-consistency losses. Its robustness dealing with data that suffer from domain-specific nonlinear deformations has been evaluated through comparison experiments performed on a multi-sequence brain MR dataset and a multi-modality abdominal dataset. Our method has displayed its ability to generate synthesized data that is aligned with the source while maintaining a proper quality of signal compared to CycleGAN-generated data. The proposed model also obtained comparable performance with CycleGAN when data from the source and target domains are alignable through simple affine transformations.

Keywords: Synthesis · Deep learning · GAN · Unsupervised learning

1 Introduction

Modern clinical practices make cross-domain medical image synthesis a technology gaining in popularity. (In this paper, we use the term "domain" to uniformly address different imaging modalities and parametric configurations.) Image synthesis allows one to handle and impute data of missing domains in standard statistical analysis [1], or to improve intermediate step of analysis such as registration [2], segmentation [3] and disease classification [4]. Our application is to

---

C. Wang—This work was supported by British Heart Foundation.

A. Gooya et al. (Eds.): SASHIMI 2018, LNCS 11037, pp. 52–60, 2018.
https://doi.org/10.1007/978-3-030-00536-8_6

generate pseudo-CT images from multi-sequence MR data [5]. The synthesized pseudo-CT images can be further used for the purpose of PET-MR attenuation correction [6].

State-of-the-art methods often train a deep convolutional neural network (CNN) as image generator following the learning procedure of the generative adversarial network (GAN) [7]. Many of these methods require to use aligned, or paired, datasets which is hard to obtain in practice when the data can not be aligned through an affine transformation. To deal with unpaired cross-domain data, a recent trend is to leverage CycleGAN losses [8] into the learning process to capture high-level information translatable between domains. Previous studies have shown that CycleGAN is robust to unpaired data [9]. However, not all information encoded in CycleGAN image generators should be used due to very distinct imaging qualities and characteristics in different domains, especially different modalities. Figure 1 displays a representative example of CycleGAN based cross-modality synthesis where the real CT and MR data were acquired from the same patient. It can be seen that the shape and relative positions of the scanner beds are very different. This problem can be addressed as "domain-specific deformation". Because the generator networks can not treat the spatial deformation and image contents separately, CycleGAN encodes this information and reproduce it in the forward pass, which causes misalignment between the source and synthesized images. For some applications, such as generating pseudo-CT for attenuation correction of PET-MR data, this domain-specific deformation should be discarded. In the mean time, the networks should keep efficient information about appearences of the same anatomy in distinct domains. A popular strategy to solve this problem is performing supervised or semi-supervised learning with an extra mission, for example, segmentation [10], but this requires collection of extra ground truth.

In this paper, we present a deformation invariant CycleGAN (DicycleGAN) framework for cross-domain medical image synthesis. The architecture of the networks is inspired by the design of deformable convolutional network (DCN) [11]. We handle the different nonlinear deformations in different domains by integrating a modified DCN structure into the image generators and propose to use normalized mutual information (NMI) in the CycleGAN loss. We evaluate the proposed network using both multi-modality abdominal aortic data and multi-sequence brain MR data. The experimental results demonstrate the ability of our method to handle highly disparate imaging domains and generate synthesized images aligned with the source data. In the mean time, the quality of the synthesized images are as good as those generated by the CycleGAN model. The main contributions of this paper include a new DicycleGAN architecture which learns deformation-invariant correspondences between domains and a new NMI-based cycleGAN loss.

Table 1. Synthesis results of IXI dataset using undeformed T2 images.

Experiment	Model	MSE	PSNR	SSIM
PD to T2	Cycle	0.186 (0.08)	**27.35 (1.69)**	0.854 (0.03)
	Dicycle	**0.183 (0.09)**	26.49 (1.62)	**0.871 (0.03)**
T2 to PD	Cycle	**0.134 (0.02)**	**29.68 (1.61)**	**0.892 (0.03)**
	Dicycle	0.146 (0.03)	28.85 (1.59)	0.883 (0.02)

2   Method

A GAN framework using a image generator G to synthesize images of a target domain using images from a source domain, and a discriminator D to distinguish real and synthesized images. Parameters of G are optimized to confuse D, while D is trained at the same time for better binary classification performance to classify real and synthesized data. We assumes that we have n^A images $x^A \in \mathcal{X}^A$ from domain $\mathcal{X}^A$, and n^B images $x^B \in \mathcal{X}^B$. To generate synthesized images of domain $\mathcal{X}^B$ using images from $\mathcal{X}^A$, G and D are trained in the min-max game of the GAN loss $\mathcal{L}_{GAN}\left(G, D, \mathcal{X}^A, \mathcal{X}^B\right)$ [7]. When dealing with unpaired data, the original CycleGAN framework consists of two symmetric sets of generators $G^{A \to B}$ and $G^{B \to A}$ act as mapping functions applied to a source domain, and two discriminators D^B and D^A to distinguish real and synthesized data for a target domain. The *cycle consistency* loss $\mathcal{L}_{cyc}\left(G^{A \to B}, D^A, G^{B \to A}, D^B, \mathcal{X}^A, \mathcal{X}^B\right)$, or $\mathcal{L}_{cyc}^{A,B}$, is used to keep the cycle-consistency between the two sets of networks. The loss of the whole CycleGAN framework $\mathcal{L}_{CycleGAN} = \mathcal{L}_{GAN}^{A \to B} + \mathcal{L}_{GAN}^{B \to A} + \lambda_{cyc}\mathcal{L}_{cyc}^{A,B}$. (In this paper we use the short expression $\mathcal{L}_{GAN}^{A \to B}$ to denote GAN loss $\mathcal{L}_{GAN}(G^{A \to B}, D^B, \mathcal{X}^A, \mathcal{X}^B)$). The image generator in the CycleGAN contains an input convolutional block, two down-sampling convolutional layers, followed by a few resnet blocks or a Unet structure, and two up-sampling transpose convolutional blocks before the last two convolutional blocks.

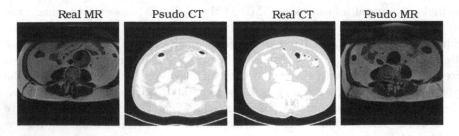

| Real MR | Psudo CT | Real CT | Psudo MR |

Fig. 1. Example of MR-CT synthesis using vanila CycleGAN.

DicycleGAN Architecture. In order to capture deformation-invariant information between domains, we introduce a modified DCN architecture into the image generators of CycleGAN, as shown in Fig. 2. The deformable convolution can be viewed as an atrous convolution kernel with trainable dilation rates and reinterpolated input feature map [11]. The spatial offsets of each point in the feature map is learned through a conventional convolution operation, followed by another convolution layer. This leads to a "Lasagne" structure consist of interleaved "offset convolution" and conventional convolution operations. We adopt this structure to the generators by inserting an offset convolutional operation (displayed in cyan in Fig. 2) in front of the input convolutional block, downsample convolutional blocks and the first resnet blocks. Note that this "offset" convolution only affects the interpolation of the input feature map rather than providing a real convolution result. Let θ_T denote the learnable parameters in the "offset" convolutional layers, and θ the rest parameters in image generator G. When training G, each input image x generates two output images: deformed output image $G_T(x) = G(x|\theta, \theta_T)$ and undeformed image $G(x) = G(x|\theta)$. The red and blue arrows in Fig. 2 indicate the computation flows for generating $G_T(x)$ and $G(x)$ in the forward passes. $G_T(x)$ is then taken by the corresponding discriminator D for calculation of GAN losses, and $G(x)$ is expected to be aligned with x.

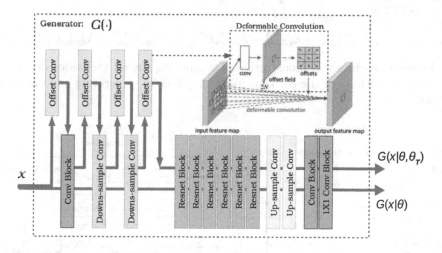

Fig. 2. Architecture of the proposed image generator $G(\cdot)$. Each input image x generates a deformed output $G(x|\theta, \theta_T)$ and an undeformed output $G(x|\theta)$ through two forward passes shown in red and blue. Demonstration of deformable convolution is obtained from [11]. (best viewed in color)

DicycleGAN Loss. DicycleGAN loss contains traditional GAN loss following the implementation of CycleGAN [8], but also includes an image alignment loss and a new cycle consistency loss. For the GAN loss $L_{GAN}^{A \to B}$, the image generator $G^{A \to B}$ is trained to minimize $\left(D^B\left(G_T^{A \to B}\left(x^A\right)\right) - 1\right)^2$ and D^B is trained to minimize $\left(D^B(x^B) - 1\right)^2 + D^B \left(G_T^{A \to B}(x^A)\right)^2$. The same formulation is used to calculate $\mathcal{L}_{GAN}^{B \to A}$ defined on $G^{B \to A}$ and D^A. Note that the GAN loss is calculated based on the deformed synthesized images. As the undeformed outputs of generators are expected to be aligned with the input images, we propose to use a information loss based on normalized mutual information (NMI). NMI is a popular metric used for image registration. It varies between 0 and 1 indicating alignment of two clustered images [12]. The image alignment loss is defined as:

$$\mathcal{L}_{align}^{A,B} = 2 - NMI\left(x^A, G^{A \to B}\left(x^A\right)\right) - NMI\left(x^B, G^{B \to A}\left(x^B\right)\right). \quad (1)$$

Based on the proposed design of image generators, the cycle two types of cycle consistency losses. The undeformed cycle consistency loss is defined as:

$$\mathcal{L}_{cyc}^{A,B} = \|G^{B \to A}\left(G^{A \to B}\left(x^A\right)\right) - x^A\|_1 + \|G^{A \to B}\left(G^{B \to A}\left(x^B\right)\right) - x^B\|_1. \quad (2)$$

Beside $\mathcal{L}_{cyc}$, the deformation applied to the synthesized image should be also cycle consistent. Here we defined a deformation-invariant cycle consistency loss:

$$\mathcal{L}_{dicyc}^{A,B} = \|G_T^{B \to A}\left(G_T^{A \to B}\left(x^A\right)\right) - x^A\|_1 + \|G_T^{A \to B}\left(G_T^{B \to A}\left(x^B\right)\right) - x^B\|_1. \quad (3)$$

To perform image synthesis between domains $\mathcal{X}^A$ and $\mathcal{X}^B$, we use the deformed output images $G_T^{A \to B}$ and $G_T^{B \to A}$ to calculate the GAN loss. The full loss of DicycleGAN is:

$$\mathcal{L}_{DicycleGAN} = \mathcal{L}_{GAN}^{A \to B} + \mathcal{L}_{GAN}^{B \to A} + \lambda_{align}\mathcal{L}_{align}^{A,B} + \lambda_{cyc}\mathcal{L}_{cyc}^{A,B} + \lambda_{dicyc}\mathcal{L}_{dicyc}^{A,B}. \quad (4)$$

Figure 3 provides a demonstration of computing the all the losses discussed above using outputs of the corresponding DicycleGAN generators and discriminators.

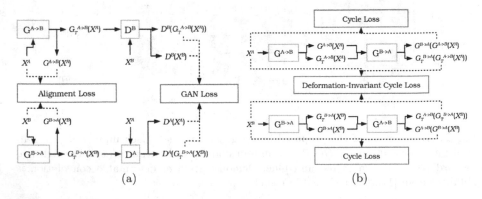

(a)   (b)

Fig. 3. Calculation of losses in DicycleGAN. (a) shows GAN and image alignment losses: the undeformed output of the image generators are used for alignment losses, and the deformed outputs for GAN losses. (b) shows the Cycle consistency losses.

3   Experiments

Evaluation Metrics. The most widely used quantitative evaluation metrics for cross-domain image synthesis are: mean squared error (MSE), peak signal-to-noise ratio (PSNR) and structural similarity index (SSIM). Given a volume x^A and a target volume x^B, the MSE is computed as: $\frac{1}{N}\sum_1^N \left(x^B - G^{A\to B}(x^A)\right)^2$, where N is number of voxels in the volume. PSNR is calculated as: $10\log_{10}\frac{\max_B^2}{MSE}$. SSIM is computed as: $\frac{(2\mu_A\mu_B+c_1)(2\delta_{AB}+c2)}{(\mu_A^2+\mu_B^2+c_1)(\delta_A^2+\delta+B^2+c2)}$, where μ and δ^2 are mean and variance of a volume, and δ_{AB} is the covariance between x^A and x^B. c_1 and c_2 are two variables to stabilize the division with weak denominator [13].

Datasets. We use the Information eXtraction from Images (IXI) dataset[1] which provides co-registered multi-sequence skull-stripped MR images collected from multiple sites. Due to the limited storage space, here we selected 66 proton density (PD-) and T2-weighted volumes, each volume contains 116 to 130 2D slices. We use 38 pairs for training and 28 pairs for evaluation of synthesis results. Our image generators take 2D axial-plane slices of the volumes as inputs. During the training phase, we resample all volumes to a resolution of $1.8 \times 1.8 \times 1.8\,\mathrm{mm}^3/voxel$, then crop the volumes to 128×128 pixel images. As the generators in both Cycle-GAN and DicycleGAN are fully convolutional, the predictions are performed on full size images. All the images are normalized with their mean and standard deviation. We also used a private dataset contains 40 multi-modality abdominal T2*-weighted images and CT images collected from 20 patients with abdominal aortic aneurysm (AAA) in a clinical trial. All images are resampled to a resolution of $1.56 \times 1.56 \times 5\,\mathrm{mm}^3/voxel$, and the axial-plane slices trimmed to 192×192 pixels. It is difficult to non-rigidly register whole abdominal images to calculate the evaluation metrics, but the aorta can be rigidly aligned to assess the performance of image synthesis. The anatomy of the aorta have previously been co-registered and segmented by 4 clinical researchers.

Implementation Details. We used image generators with 9 Resnet blocks. All parameters of, or inherit from, vanilla CycleGAN are taken from the original paper. For the DicycleGAN, we set $\lambda_{cyc} = \lambda_{dicyc} = 10$ and $\lambda_{align} = 0.9$. The models were trained with Adam optimizer [14] with a fixed learning rate of 0.0002 for the first 100 epochs, followed by 100 epochs with linearly decreasing learning rate. Here we apply a simple early stop strategy: in the first 100 epochs, when $\mathcal{L}_{DicycleGAN}$ stops decreasing for 10 epochs, the training will move to the learning rate decaying stage; this tolerance is set to 20 epochs in the second 100 epochs.

Experiments Setup. In order to quantitatively evaluate robustness of our model to the domain-specific local distortion, we applied an arbitrary non-linear distortion to the T2-weighted images of IXI. Synthesis experiments were performed between the PD-weighted data and undeformed, as well as the deformed

---

[1] http://brain-development.org/ixi-dataset/.

T2-weighted data. When using deformed T2-weighted images, the ground truth were generated by applying the same nonlinear deformation to the source PD-weighted images. We trained the CycleGAN and DicycleGAN using unpaired, randomly selected slices. The training images were augmented using aggressive flips, rotations, shearing and translations so that CycleGAN can be robust. In the test stage, the three metrics introduced above were computed. For our private dataset, the metrics were computed within the segmented aortic anatomy excluding any other imaged objects because all the three metrics require to be calculated on aligned images.

4   Results

Tables 1 and 2 present the PD-T2 co-synthesis results using undeformed and deformed T2-weighted images. In addition, Fig. 4 provides an example showing the synthesized images generated by CycleGAN and DicycleGAN. CycleGAN encoded the simulated domain-specific deformation, whether applied to source or target domain, and combined this deformation into the synthesized images. This leads to misalignment of source and synthesized images. The quantitative results show that our DicycleGAN model produced comparable results with CycleGAN when there is no domain-specific distortions, but it achieved remarkable performance gain when the source and target images can not be aligned through an affine transformation. This is because of the deformed synthesized images generated by CycleGAN which lead to severe misalignments between the source and synthesized images.

The cross-modality synthesis results are shown in Table 3. The discrepancy between the two imaging modalities can be shown by the different relative positions between the imaged objects and the beds. CycleGAN encoded this information in the image generators as shown earlier in Fig. 1.

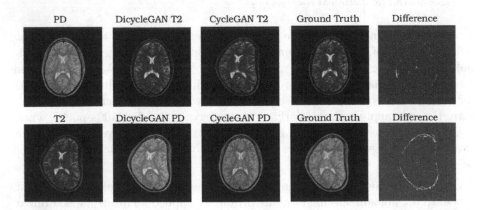

Fig. 4. Example of synthesized images generated by CycleGAN and DicycleGAN, compared to the ground truths. The ground truth of the deformed source image is generated by applying the same arbitrary deformation to the original target image.

Table 2. Synthesis results of IXI dataset using deformed T2 images.

Experiment	Model	MSE	PSNR	SSIM
PD to T2	Cycle	0.586 (0.25)	19.52 (1.62)	0.6081 (0.12)
	Dicycle	**0.145 (0.02)**	**22.32 (1.29)**	**0.7842 (0.03)**
T2 to PD	Cycle	0.561 (0.22)	19.42 (1.61)	0.6001 (0.11)
	Dicycle	**0.141 (0.02)**	**22.86 (1.31)**	**0.7714 (0.02)**

Table 3. Multi-modality synthesis results using private dataset.

Experiment	Model	MSE	PSNR	SSIM
T2* to CT	Cycle	0.516 (0.19)	18.32 (1.82)	0.5716 (0.15)
	Dicycle	**0.287 (0.11)**	**23.71 (1.17)**	**0.7122 (0.03)**
CT to T2*	Cycle	0.521 (0.22)	19.12 (1.60)	0.5818 (0.12)
	Dicycle	**0.299 (0.08)**	**22.66 (1.11)**	**0.7556 (0.02)**

5 Conclusion and Discussion

We propose a new method for cross-domain medical image synthesis, called Dicy-cleGAN. Compared to the vanilla CycleGAN method, we integrate DCN layers into the image generators and reinforce the training process with deformation-invariant cycle consistency loss and NMI-based alignment loss. Results obtained from both multi-sequence MR dataset and our private multi-modality abdominal dataset shows that our model achieved comparable performance with CycleGAN when the source and target data can be aligned with an affine transformation. Our model achieved obvious performance gain compared to CycleGAN when there are domain-specific nonlinear deformations. A possible future application of DicycleGAN is multi-modal image registration.

References

1. van Tulder, G., de Bruijne, M.: Why does synthesized data improve multi-sequence classification? In: Navab, N., Hornegger, J., Wells, W.M., Frangi, A.F. (eds.) MIC-CAI 2015. LNCS, vol. 9349, pp. 531–538. Springer, Cham (2015). https://doi.org/10.1007/978-3-319-24553-9_65
2. Iglesias, J.E., Konukoglu, E., Zikic, D., Glocker, B., Van Leemput, K., Fischl, B.: Is synthesizing MRI contrast useful for inter-modality analysis? In: Mori, K., Sakuma, I., Sato, Y., Barillot, C., Navab, N. (eds.) MICCAI 2013. LNCS, vol. 8149, pp. 631–638. Springer, Heidelberg (2013). https://doi.org/10.1007/978-3-642-40811-3_79
3. Roy, S., Carass, A., Prince, J.: A compressed sensing approach for MR tissue contrast synthesis. In: Székely, G., Hahn, H.K. (eds.) IPMI 2011. LNCS, vol. 6801, pp. 371–383. Springer, Heidelberg (2011). https://doi.org/10.1007/978-3-642-22092-0_31

4. Li, R., et al.: Deep learning based imaging data completion for improved brain disease diagnosis. In: Golland, P., Hata, N., Barillot, C., Hornegger, J., Howe, R. (eds.) MICCAI 2014. LNCS, vol. 8675, pp. 305–312. Springer, Cham (2014). https://doi.org/10.1007/978-3-319-10443-0_39

5. Nie, D., et al.: Medical image synthesis with context-aware generative adversarial networks. In: Descoteaux, M., Maier-Hein, L., Franz, A., Jannin, P., Collins, D.L., Duchesne, S. (eds.) MICCAI 2017. LNCS, vol. 10435, pp. 417–425. Springer, Cham (2017). https://doi.org/10.1007/978-3-319-66179-7_48

6. Wagenknecht, G., Kaiser, H.J., Mottaghy, F.M., Herzog, H.: MRI for attenuation correction in PET: methods and challenges. Magn. Resonance Mater. Phys. Biol. Med. **26**(1), 99–113 (2013)

7. Goodfellow, I., et al.: Generative adversarial nets. In: Advances in Neural Information Processing Systems, pp. 2672–2680 (2014)

8. Zhu, J.Y., Park, T., Isola, P., Efros, A.A.: Unpaired image-to-image translation using cycle-consistent adversarial networks. arXiv preprint arXiv:1703.10593 (2017)

9. Wolterink, J.M., Dinkla, A.M., Savenije, M.H.F., Seevinck, P.R., van den Berg, C.A.T., Išgum, I.: Deep MR to CT synthesis using unpaired data. In: Tsaftaris, S.A., Gooya, A., Frangi, A.F., Prince, J.L. (eds.) SASHIMI 2017. LNCS, vol. 10557, pp. 14–23. Springer, Cham (2017). https://doi.org/10.1007/978-3-319-68127-6_2

10. Huo, Y., Xu, Z., Bao, S., Assad, A., Abramson, R.G., Landman, B.A.: Adversarial synthesis learning enables segmentation without target modality ground truth. arXiv preprint arXiv:1712.07695 (2017)

11. Dai, J., et al.: Deformable convolutional networks. CoRR, abs/1703.06211 **1**(2), 3 (2017)

12. Vinh, N.X., Epps, J., Bailey, J.: Information theoretic measures for clusterings comparison: variants, properties, normalization and correction for chance. J. Mach. Learn. Res. **11**(Oct), 2837–2854 (2010)

13. Larkin, K.G.: Structural similarity index SSIMplified (2015)

14. Kingma, D.P., Ba, J.: Adam: a method for stochastic optimization. arXiv preprint arXiv:1412.6980 (2014)

Deep Boosted Regression for MR to CT Synthesis

Kerstin Kläser[1]([✉]), Pawel Markiewicz[1], Marta Ranzini[1], Wenqi Li[2],
Marc Modat[1,2], Brian F. Hutton[3], David Atkinson[4], Kris Thielemans[3],
M. Jorge Cardoso[1,2], and Sébastien Ourselin[2]

[1] Centre for Medical Image Computing, University College London, London, UK
kerstin.klaser.16@ucl.ac.uk
[2] School of Biomedical Engineering and Imaging Sciences,
King's College London, London, UK
[3] Institute of Nuclear Medicine, University College London, London, UK
[4] Centre for Medical Imaging, University College London, London, UK

Abstract. Attenuation correction is an essential requirement of positron emission tomography (PET) image reconstruction to allow for accurate quantification. However, attenuation correction is particularly challenging for PET-MRI as neither PET nor magnetic resonance imaging (MRI) can directly image tissue attenuation properties. MRI-based computed tomography (CT) synthesis has been proposed as an alternative to physics based and segmentation-based approaches that assign a population-based tissue density value in order to generate an attenuation map. We propose a novel deep fully convolutional neural network that generates synthetic CTs in a recursive manner by gradually reducing the residuals of the previous network, increasing the overall accuracy and generalisability, while keeping the number of trainable parameters within reasonable limits. The model is trained on a database of 20 pre-acquired MRI/CT pairs and a four-fold random bootstrapped validation with a 80:20 split is performed. Quantitative results show that the proposed framework outperforms a state-of-the-art atlas-based approach decreasing the Mean Absolute Error (MAE) from 131HU to 68HU for the synthetic CTs and reducing the PET reconstruction error from 14.3% to 7.2%.

1 Introduction

Positron emission tomography - magnetic resonance imaging (PET-MRI) is a relatively new joint imaging technique that combines the functional information from PET with the flexibility of MRI. To obtain quantitative PET images, it is essential to know the tissue attenuation coefficients throughout the patient. However, this is a difficult problem for PET-MRI as neither PET nor MRI can directly image tissue attenuation properties, which is why computer tomography (CT) remains the clinically accepted gold-standard for attenuation correction. However, it is desirable to circumvent the requirement of an additional CT acquisition not just to reduce the exposed radiation dose to the patient but also to

© Springer Nature Switzerland AG 2018
A. Gooya et al. (Eds.): SASHIMI 2018, LNCS 11037, pp. 61–70, 2018.
https://doi.org/10.1007/978-3-030-00536-8_7

avoid the risk of registration errors between the MR and CT volumes. Hence, synthesising pseudo CTs from MR images gained a lot of interest in the field of attenuation correction for hybrid PET-MR systems.

Within the last ten years, several research groups focused on the development of single- and multi-atlas-based approaches that predict attenuation coefficients on a continuous scale by deforming an anatomical model or dataset to match the subject's anatomy using non-rigid registration. Synthesis methods based on multi-atlas information propagation, such as the model proposed by Burgos et al. [1], have dominated this area of research for several years.

Recently, deep learning approaches have started outperforming multi-atlas methods. In particular, convolutional neural networks (CNNs) have proved to be a powerful tool for translating an image between domains (as between MRI and CT). Within deep learning approaches, methods for image-to-image translation can be classified into two classes: unsupervised and supervised representation learning. The first learns the contextual information between two image domains from unpaired data, allowing general-purpose image-to-image translation. For example, Zhu et al. recently proposed a CycleGAN model that assumes an underlying relationship between two different domains that can be learned by an adversarial loss that competes with a second network trained to produce images that are in principle indistinguishable from the desired output [2]. Recently, Wolternik et al. successfully applied the CycleGAN model to medical image data in order to perform CT synthesis [3]. However, just like the majority of CNN frameworks, their framework addresses the image translation problem on the basis of 2D image representations, neglecting the 3 dimensional nature of the anatomical representation. Several attempts have been made to stably train 3 dimensional networks, a challenging task due to the curse of dimensionality. Most 3D network architectures exploit a fully convolutional architecture, where neighbourhood information is preserved either through pooling/upsampling layers [4,5], or through the use of dilated convolutions [6]. Here, we approach the image translation task in a supervised learning setting, where corresponding data pairs are available. However, unlike previous supervised methods [7], we propose to use a fully 3D architecture with an efficient parameter count and large receptive field, namely HighRes3DNet by Li et al. [6], to learn a 3 dimensional representation of the data. This representation is then mapped to the domain of CT images through a series of 1D convolutions with non-linear activation functions. This proposed architecture also makes extensive use of residual connections to avoid the need to model the identity mapping of the representation, improving the overall accuracy and training stability. Finally, we reformulate the residual connection architecture as a corrective model, which can be seen as a form of boosting in classic machine learning. This is achieved by recursively applying a corrective model with shared parameters and with a deep supervision loss, recursively reducing the residuals of the predictions. We evaluate our approach on a dataset of 20 patients using a four-fold random bootstrapped validation with a 80:20 split. The results demonstrate an improvement over a state-of-the-art multi-atlas based method, as well as the ability of our method to simulate abnormal structures not observable in the training data. As we are validating the advantages of the use of a recursive boosting model, the contribution of the paper is independent of the choice of cost function.

2   Methods

2.1   Deep Boosted Regression

The aim of the proposed image synthesis approach is to find a mapping from the domain of T1- and T2-weighted MR input images to the domain of CT images. This mapping can be formulated as

$$\mathbb{R}^{T_1, T_2} \rightarrow \mathbb{R}^{CT},$$

which is a mapping from $y \hookleftarrow f(x)$, where f is a function that maps input $x \in \mathbb{R}^{T_1, T_2}$ to $y \in \mathbb{R}^{CT}$. This mapping function is highly nonlinear, and can be approximated by a composition of simpler functions with parameters ϕ, of the form $\tilde{y} = f^{(n)}(f^{(n-1)}(\dots(f^{(2)}(f^{(1)}(x, \phi_1), \phi_2), \dots), \phi_{n-1}), \phi_n)$. In a supervised learning context, these parameters ϕ are determined by minimising a loss function that aims to minimise the residuals between the predicted CT $\tilde{y}$ and the true CT y

$$\mathcal{L}_2 = ||y - \tilde{y}||_2$$

Note, however, that the large number of functions and parameters ϕ creates computational and optimisation challenges. To avoid this, we propose to formulate the problem as a boosting model, where the output of each function $f^{(n)}$ aims to approximate y. If $\tilde{y}_1 = f^{(1)}(x, \phi_1)$, then subsequent functions can be seen as a form of corrective learning, as $\tilde{y}_2 = f^{(2)}(\tilde{y}_1, x)$. Thus, the model above can be rewritten as

$$\tilde{y} = f^{(n)}(f^{(n-1)}(\dots(f^{(2)}(f^{(1)}(x, \phi_1), x, \phi_2), \dots), x, \phi_{n-1}), x, \phi_n).$$

It is important to note that this corrective learning model introduces more parameters for every corrective function f, resulting in model overfit and making it hard to optimise. Instead, we propose to create a single corrective function $f^{(c)}$, equivalent to sharing parameters between functions $f^{(2)}$ to $f^{(n)}$, which is applied recursively after an initial approximation of $\tilde{y}$ given by $f^{(1)}$. We can define our recursion as

$$\tilde{y}_k = \begin{cases} f^{(1)}(x \mid N_1) & if \ k = 0 \\ f^{(c)}(x, \tilde{y}_{k-1} \mid N_c) & if \ k > 0 \end{cases}$$

where a function with parameters N_1 synthesises $\tilde{y}_1$ from an input MRI x, at iteration $k = 0$. For $k > 0$, a corrective function, with parameters N_c, maps the previous prediction $\tilde{y}_{k-1}$ and the input MR images x to a better approximation of the true CT y. Finally, to ensure that the function's parameters can be optimised, we change the loss function to

$$Loss = \sum_{k=0}^{n} \|\tilde{y}_k - y\|^2.$$

thus providing a form of deep supervision by introducing gradients for each function f. We called this method Deep Boosted Regression as it is inspired by the recursive residual minimisation approach of classical boosting models.

2.2 Proposed Network Architecture

The functions described in the previous section are approximated by two separate CNNs, both following the network architecture of the high-resolution compact architecture presented by Li et al. [6], which has been shown to be very efficient in learning 3D representations from large-scale image data. It consists of 20 convolutional layers with kernel size $3 \times 3 \times 3$ that encode low-level image features. Mid- and high-level image features are captured within the following convolutional layers with kernels that are dilated by a factor of two or four, respectively, preserving the spatial resolution of the input image throughout the network. Convolutional layers are grouped into pairs of two, and residual connections are added that enable an identity mapping so that both parameters and computational cost are minimal as shown by He et al. [8].

The proposed network architecture is illustrated in Fig. 1. The first network N_1 is trained to synthesise an initial pseudo CT (pCT) taking both T1- and T2-weighted MR images as inputs. This first pCT is passed to a second network N_c that learns the residuals between pCT and the real CT. Therefore the weights of N_c depend on the output of N_1, but not vice versa. An improved pCT is then generated by adding the residuals to the initially synthesised pCT, which is then again fed back into N_c in order to update the weights of the network. By sharing the parameters of N_c no additional parameters are introduced to the network keeping computational complexity within limits and making the model more generalisable even if only a limited number of training datasets are available. This recursive cycle can be repeated for k iterations, however, the number of iterations is limited to avoid overfitting. The proposed Deep Boosted Regression (DBR) approach exploits the advantages of the recursive boosting model and is therefore independent of the choice of the cost function.

2.3 Implementation Details

In the training stage, the data (see Sect. 3) were randomly sampled into subvolumes of size $56 \times 56 \times 56$ pixels that were augmented by randomly rotating each of the three orthogonal planes on the fly by an angle in the interval of $[-10°, 10°]$. The MR data was also randomly scaled by a factor between 0.9 and 1.1. Patches were sampled more often from high frequency regions of the image as these areas are harder to model. The network was trained from scratch on a

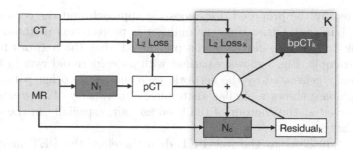

Fig. 1. Framework of proposed Deep Boosted Regression method. MRs are fed into a first network N_1, an initial pseudo CT (pCT) is synthesised by minimising the loss between pCT and original CT. Within the space K, residual learning is performed, where the residuals are added to pCT and fed into a second network N_c, wherefore the "+" illustrates an accumulator. A second loss is introduced minimising the difference between ground-truth CT and updated pCT. The final output is an error boosted pCT (bpCT). The number of residual learning cycles (K) is limited to avoid overfitting (e.g. we used K = 4).

single NVIDIA Titan X GPU using the Adam optimisation method. We did a four-fold random bootstrapped validation, where for each fold, the data was split into 70% training, 10% validation and 20% testing data. The model was trained with a learning rate of 0.001 and a weight decay of 5.0×10^{-8}. We trained the network for 10K iterations before decreasing the learning rate by a factor of 10. We terminated the training after 40K iterations when the error had converged. The training and validation loss is demonstrated in Fig. 2. We implemented our method with NiftyNet, which is a TensorFlow-based open-source CNN platform that can be used for research in medical image analysis. The model will be made available online as part of the NiftyNet model zoo [9].

3   Experimental Datasets and Materials

The experimental dataset consisted of pairs of T1- and T2-weighted MR and CT brain images of 20 patients. For each subject MRs and CTs were aligned using first a rigid registration algorithm followed by a very low degree of freedom non-rigid deformation [1]. A second non-linear registration was performed, using a cubic B-spline with normalised mutual information, only on the neck region to correct for soft tissue shift [10]. Each volume had $301 \times 301 \times 153$ voxels with a voxel size of approximately $1\,\text{mm}^3$. For evaluation purposes a head region mask was extracted from the CT image to exclude the background from the analysis.

4   Experiments and Results

Figure 3 shows an example MR input image, a synthesised CT image obtained by a current state-of-the-art multi-atlas propagation approach [1], a synthesised

CT generated by the proposed deep boosting approach and the corresponding reference CT images. Other than the multi-atlas propagation method, our network is able to generate details in the pseudo CT that the network has never seen. For example, Fig. 3 shows a patient with an epidermoid cyst in the skull being correctly generated by the network, even though no other patient in the training database shows a similar anatomical abnormality. The greatest error can be observed at the contour of the head and air, especially in the region of the nasal cavity.

We had no access to the raw PET data therefore the PET images were reconstructed using the following simulation using NiftyPET software [11]. The original PET image was forward projected using the Siemens mMR scanner geometry, then multiplied by the forward projected CT-based attenuation map in order to obtain simulated measured PET sinograms. The simulated measured data were then reconstructed using the original CT-based attenuation map to obtain a reference image, to which the reconstructed images obtained by the multi-atlas propagation method and our Deep Boosted Regression approach were compared. Figure 4 shows an example slice of the simulated reference PET, the synthesised PET and the corresponding difference image generated by the multi-atlas propagation method and the proposed DBR approach, respectively.

In order to quantify the results we calculated the Mean Absolute Error (MAE) of the synthesised CTs only within the head region by masking the

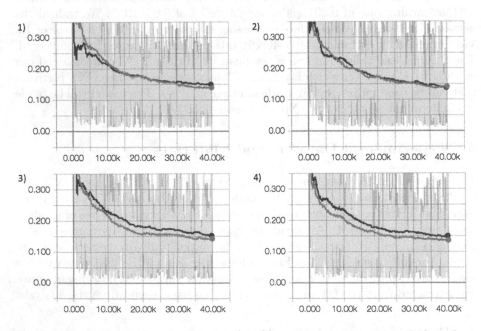

Fig. 2. Training (orange) and validation (blue) loss for each fold of four-fold random bootstrapped validation with a 80:20 split. The training was terminated after 40K iterations when the error had converged. (Color figure online)

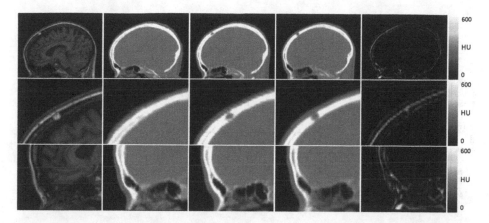

Fig. 3. From left to right: Input MR image, synthesised CT using multi-atlas propagation approach, reference real CT, synthesised CT using proposed Deep Boosted Regression, and absolute error between real and synthesised boosted CT images of the whole head (top), an anatomical abnormality in the skull (middle) and the sinus region (bottom).

surrounding air out and compared it to the multi-atlas propagation method. The choice of MAE as error metric derives from its good suitability for PET attenuation correction and due to the quantitative nature of CT images. We also investigated how the MAE of the testing data progresses after each run through the network. The results are demonstrated in Fig. 5. The average MAE of the test images synthesised with the multi-atlas propagation approach lies around 131.4HU, whereas the proposed method for MR-to-CT translation is able to reduce this error by around 48%. A paired t-test was used to show that the agreement between true CT images and images generated by the proposed model was significantly higher ($p < 10^{-5}$) compared to the images synthesised using the multi-atlas propagation approach. The MAE also significantly reduces after the first two boosting cycles of the network confirming that the integrated boosting for the minimisation of the residuals works. Table 1 shows a direct comparison between the proposed model, the multi-atlas propagation approach and two other recent deep learning methods for MR to CT synthesis.

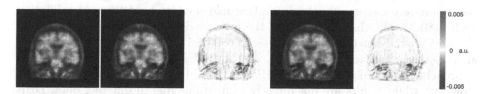

Fig. 4. From left to right: PET reconstructed with real CT, with synthesised CT using multi-atlas propagation approach (mapCT), difference between real CT and mapCT, PET reconstructed with synthesised CT from Deep Boosted Regression (bpCT), difference between real CT and bpCT.

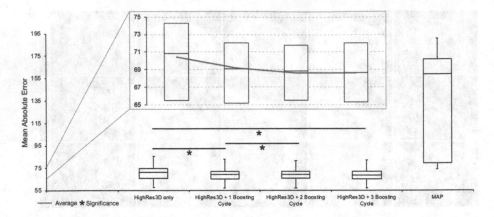

Fig. 5. Progression of Mean Absolute Error (MAE) of synthesised CTs after each step of the Deep Boosted Regression network (zoomed panel) compared to a current state-of-the-art multi-atlas propagation method (MAP). The MAE decreases significantly after the first and second boosting cycle (horizontal lines with asterisk) as well as overall compared to a simple feed forward network (HighRes3D only).

Table 1. Mean absolute error (MAE) in Houndsfield Units (HU) of state-of-the-art multi-atlas propagation method, two deep learning CT synthesis methods and proposed Deep Boosted Regression

Method	Mean Absolute Error
Multi-atlas propagation [1]	131.4HU ± 60HU
Context-aware generative adversarial network [12]	92.5HU ± 13.9HU
Deep CNN [7]	84.8HU ± 17.3HU
Deep Boosted Regression	68.6HU ± 15HU

5 Discussion and Conclusion

In this work we proposed a new image-to-image translation network that is able to synthesise CT images from input MR images by gradually reducing the error using a separate boosting network. We validated the advantages of the recursive boosting model using a four-fold random bootstrapped validation with a 80:20 split that showed that the average difference between synthesised CT and ground-truth CT images was 68.6HU ± 15HU, compared to Burgos et al.'s method that achieved a MAE of 131.4HU ± 60HU. Other deep learning approaches reported a MAE of 92.5HU ± 13.9HU [12] and 84.8HU ± 17.3HU [7]. However, while results are not directly comparable due to differing data, DBR reports state-of-the-art results on MAE among other deep learning approaches.

To quantify the performance of the proposed Deep Boosted Regression method relative to the CT-based attenuation correction, the mean absolute percentage error (MAPE) within the head region only was used as the figure of merit. The obtained MAPE for the proposed method was 7.2%, which showed an improvement to the state-of-the-art method [1], which obtained MAPE of 14.3%. As part of our future work, we will also investigate the impact of the synthesised CT images in radiotherapy treatment dose planning.

Furthermore, the success of the training highly depends on the registration quality of the MR/CT database. Even small inaccuracies in the registration can have a great influence on the training. An idea to circumvent the requirement of paired data is to incorporate a generative adversarial loss which provides a means of learning the context between CT and MR images from unpaired data. This has potential to provide a significant advantage in terms of the data availability for training due to the scarcity of accurately paired datasets, however, challenges in terms of validation emerge due to a missing ground truth. Moreover, we intend to extend the weighted patch sampling scheme to an adaptive sampling scheme that samples patches dynamically from areas with large residuals.

Acknowledgments. This work was supported by an IMPACT studentship funded jointly by Siemens and the EPSRC UCL Centre for Doctoral Training in Medical Imaging (EP/L016478/1). The research was also supported through the UK NIHR UCLH Biomedical Research Centre.

References

1. Burgos, N., et al.: Attenuation correction synthesis for hybrid pet-mr scanners: application to brain studies. IEEE Trans. Med. Imaging **33**(12), 2332–2341 (2014)
2. Zhu, J.Y., Park, T., Isola, P., Efros, A.A.: Unpaired image-to-image translation using cycle-consistent adversarial networks (2017). arXiv preprint arXiv:1703.10593
3. Wolterink, J.M., Dinkla, A.M., Savenije, M.H.F., Seevinck, P.R., van den Berg, C.A.T., Išgum, I.: Deep MR to CT synthesis using unpaired data. In: Tsaftaris, S.A., Gooya, A., Frangi, A.F., Prince, J.L. (eds.) SASHIMI 2017. LNCS, vol. 10557, pp. 14–23. Springer, Cham (2017). https://doi.org/10.1007/978-3-319-68127-6_2
4. Kamnitsas, K., et al.: Efficient multi-scale 3D CNN with fully connected CRF for accurate brain lesion segmentation. Med. Image Anal. **36**, 61–78 (2017)
5. Kleesiek, J., et al.: Deep MRI brain extraction: a 3D convolutional neural network for skull stripping. NeuroImage **129**, 460–469 (2016)
6. Li, W., Wang, G., Fidon, L., Ourselin, S., Cardoso, M.J., Vercauteren, T.: On the compactness, efficiency, and representation of 3D convolutional networks: brain parcellation as a pretext task. In: Niethammer, M., et al. (eds.) IPMI 2017. LNCS, vol. 10265, pp. 348–360. Springer, Cham (2017). https://doi.org/10.1007/978-3-319-59050-9_28
7. Han, X.: MR-based synthetic CT generation using a deep convolutional neural network method. Med. Phys. **44**(4), 1408–1419 (2017)
8. He, K., Zhang, X., Ren, S., Sun, J.: Deep residual learning for image recognition. CoRR abs/1512.03385 (2015)
9. Gibson, E., et al.: NiftyNet: a deep-learning platform for medical imaging. CoRR abs/1709.03485 (2017)
10. Modat, M., et al.: Fast free-form deformation using graphics processing units. Comput. Methods Prog. Biomed. **98**(3), 278–284 (2010)

11. Markiewicz, P.J., et al.: NiftyPET: a high-throughput software platform for high quantitative accuracy and precision PET imaging and analysis. Neuroinformatics **16**(1), 95–115 (2018)
12. Nie, D., et al.: Medical image synthesis with context-aware generative adversarial networks. In: Descoteaux, M., Maier-Hein, L., Franz, A., Jannin, P., Collins, D.L., Duchesne, S. (eds.) MICCAI 2017. LNCS, vol. 10435, pp. 417–425. Springer, Cham (2017). https://doi.org/10.1007/978-3-319-66179-7_48

Model-Based Generation of Synthetic 3D Time-Lapse Sequences of Multiple Mutually Interacting Motile Cells with Filopodia

Igor Peterlík[1,5], David Svoboda[2], Vladimír Ulman[3], Dmitry V. Sorokin[4], and Martin Maška[2(✉)]

[1] Institute of Computer Science, Masaryk University, Brno, Czech Republic
[2] Centre for Biomedical Image Analysis, Masaryk University, Brno, Czech Republic
xmaska@fi.muni.cz
[3] Max Planck Institute of Molecular Cell Biology and Genetics, Dresden, Germany
[4] Laboratory of Mathematical Methods of Image Processing,
Faculty of Computational Mathematics and Cybernetics,
Lomonosov Moscow State University, Moscow, Russia
[5] Inria Grand-Est, Nancy, France

Abstract. Complementing collections of 3D time-lapse image data with comprehensive manual annotations is an extremely laborious and often impracticable task, which hinders objective benchmarking of bioimage analysis workflows as well as training of widespread deep-learning-based approaches. In this paper, we present a novel simulation system capable of generating synthetic 3D time-lapse sequences of multiple mutually interacting cells with filopodial protrusions, accompanied by inherently generated reference annotations, in order to stimulate the development of fully 3D bioimage analysis workflows for filopodium segmentation and tracking in complex scenarios with multiple mutually interacting cells. The system integrates its predecessor, which was designed for single-cell, collision-unaware scenarios only, with proactive, mechanics-based handling of collisions between multiple filopodia, multiple cell bodies, or their combinations. We demonstrate its potential on two generated 3D time-lapse sequences of multiple lung cancer cells with curvilinear filopodia, which visually resemble confocal fluorescence microscopy image data.

Keywords: Simulation · 3D time-lapse sequence · Cell deformation
Cell interaction · Filopodia

1 Introduction

The imaging of cell migration and inter-cellular interactions is essential to understand various physiological and pathological processes, such as tissue morphogenesis, wound healing, embryonic development, and cancer extravasation [2,8,9]. A remarkable role in these processes involving cell interactions is attributed to

© Springer Nature Switzerland AG 2018
A. Gooya et al. (Eds.): SASHIMI 2018, LNCS 11037, pp. 71–79, 2018.
https://doi.org/10.1007/978-3-030-00536-8_8

filopodia. These are cell membrane protrusions driven by dynamic bundles of aligned actin filaments, with not fully revealed detailed biology [10,25].

The modern optical microscopy and fluorescent reporters facilitate observations of filopodial formation and dynamics in diverse three-dimensional microenvironments at unprecedented spatio-temporal resolutions [12]. However, the lack of robust and fully automatic bioimage analysis workflows for the quantification of filopodium-mediated processes in 3D+t image data impels biologists to perform such analyses solely on 2D+t image data in daily practice [1,10,22,25].

A fundamental prerequisite to bridge this gap is the availability of diverse 3D+t image datasets, accompanied by reference annotations. Such datasets allow the bioimage analysis community to objectively benchmark developed bioimage analysis workflows. Nonetheless, they are difficult to obtain due to known subjectivity, high error-proneness, and extreme labor needed for manually annotating them [6]. Therefore, the focus has recently been put on developing simulation systems that routinely generate synthetic image data, accompanied by inherently generated reference annotations, that qualitatively and quantitatively resembles real counterparts [24]. Indeed, the synthetic image data was extensively used for benchmarking of diverse time-lapse bioimage analysis algorithms [4,23] and for training of deep-learning approaches for various bioimage analysis tasks [3,26].

In this paper, we build on a recent simulation system capable of generating 3D time-lapse sequences of single motile cells with filopodial protrusions of user-controlled structural and temporal attributes [19]. Namely, we extend this single-cell, collision-unaware system to be able to generate 3D time-lapse sequences of multiple mutually interacting motile cells. By introducing proactive, mechanics-based handling of collisions, the new system can tackle various types of cell-to-cell interactions, such as the contacts between multiple filopodia, multiple cell bodies, and their mutual combinations. Its capabilities are demonstrated by generating two synthetic 3D time-lapse sequences of two and three mutually interacting lung cancer cells with single-branch filopodia of fixed geometries, visually resembling real lung cancer cells acquired using a confocal fluorescence microscope.

2   Methods of the Simulation System

In this section, we describe our simulation system, including its overview and the methodology used for modeling deformations of multiple cells with filopodia, handling their collisions, and generating realistic, time-coherent cell textures.

2.1   System Overview

We consider a simulation of a set of cells where each cell is composed of an elastic cell body and a set of deformable filopodia of fixed geometries attached to the cell body surface. The initial geometries of the cell bodies and filopodia are generated using the *geometry module* of FiloGen [19]. As the cells move, collisions between them can naturally occur. The proposed simulation system is capable of handling collisions involving any pair of the cell components, such as two filopodia, two cell bodies, or a cell body and a filopodium, including auto-collisions which can potentially occur between two components of the same cell. Finally, the deformed cell geometries are exported in each step of the simulation and provided to the module generating time-coherent cell textures, as described in Sect. 2.4.

From the mechanical point of view, the simulation is based on *constrained dynamics* of elastic objects numerically implemented using a finite element method, with two types of constraints being modeled: *equality constraints* keep filopodia attached to the respective cell body surfaces, and *inequality constraints* guarantee non-penetration of cell components during collisions.

Each time step of the mechanical simulation involves three sequential phases: *unconstrained dynamics, collision detection,* and *collision response.* Initially, the motion of each cell component is modeled *independently* according to the Newton's law of physics, which can result in violations of both equality and inequality constraints. Therefore, the vectors of *constraint violations* are computed by a proximity-based collision detection. Finally, the mechanics of each cell component is used to compute *correction forces* from the vector of violations and these forces are applied to the cell components to reimpose the constraints.

The entire simulated system can be regarded as an efficient domain decomposition where mechanical components of a large system are coupled using Lagrange multipliers computed with the Schur complement [5, 14].

2.2   Finite Element Models of Cell Components

The dynamics of each cell component c of the simulated system is given as

$$\mathbf{M}_c \ddot{\mathbf{q}}_c = \mathbf{f}_c - \mathbf{g}_c(\mathbf{q}_c, \dot{\mathbf{q}}_c) + \mathcal{H}_c^\top \boldsymbol{\lambda} \qquad (1)$$

where $\mathbf{q}_c, \dot{\mathbf{q}}_c, \ddot{\mathbf{q}}_c$ are respectively position, velocity, and acceleration of the mesh nodes representing the deformable cell component, $\mathbf{M}_c$ is an inertia matrix, $\mathbf{f}_c$ is a vector of external forces, and $\mathbf{g}_c$ is a vector of internal elastic forces. Finally, the term $\mathcal{H}_c^\top \boldsymbol{\lambda}$ represents the mechanical constraints, with $\boldsymbol{\lambda}$ being correction forces derived from the collision response. The vector $\boldsymbol{\lambda}$ is defined in a constraint space shared by all colliding and coupled components. Therefore, it must be mapped to the component space through a generally nonlinear mapping $\mathcal{H}_c$, represented by a rectangular matrix $\mathbf{H}_c$ for simplicity. The internal forces are represented as a generally nonlinear function defined as

$$\mathbf{g}_c(\mathbf{q}_c + d\mathbf{q}_c, \dot{\mathbf{q}}_c + d\dot{\mathbf{q}}_c) \approx \mathbf{g}_c(\mathbf{q}_c, \dot{\mathbf{q}}_c) + \frac{\partial \mathbf{g}_c}{\partial \mathbf{q}} d\mathbf{q}_c + \frac{\partial \mathbf{g}_c}{\partial \dot{\mathbf{q}}} d\dot{\mathbf{q}}_c. \qquad (2)$$

Its derivatives, $\mathbf{K}_c = \frac{\partial \mathbf{g}_c}{\partial \mathbf{q}}$ and $\mathbf{B}_c = \frac{\partial \mathbf{g}_c}{\partial \dot{\mathbf{q}}}$, are known as the stiffness and damping matrices, respectively.

The system described by (1) is integrated using the Euler implicit scheme: denoting t the previous time step, the velocity update in the actual time step $t + h$ is computed as

$$\underbrace{(\mathbf{M}_c - h\mathbf{B}_c - h^2 \mathbf{K}_c)}_{\mathbf{A}_c} d\dot{\mathbf{q}}_c = \underbrace{h\mathbf{g}_c - h^2 \mathbf{K}_c \dot{\mathbf{q}}_c^t + \mathbf{f}_c}_{\mathbf{b}_c} + h\mathbf{H}_c^\top \boldsymbol{\lambda}, \qquad (3)$$

being discretized using finite element models that reflect the cell component type. Linear co-rotational beam elements based on the Tymoshenko formulation [17] are considered in the case of a filopodium φ. Organized in piecewise linear segments, its nodes $\mathbf{q}_\varphi$ have six degrees of freedom (DoFs). The stiffness matrix $\mathbf{K}_\varphi$, consisted of 12×12 blocks as each beam relates two 6-DoF nodes, is parametrized with Young's modulus E_φ, Poisson ratio ν_φ, and the beam radius r_φ. As for a cell body β, linear tetrahedral P1 elements are considered and co-rotational formulation of linear elasticity is used [11]. The nodes $\mathbf{q}_\beta$ have three DoFs and the stiffness matrix $\mathbf{K}_\beta$, consisted of 12×12 blocks relating the contributions of four 3-DoF nodes connected to a P1 element, is parametrized with Young's modulus E_β and Poisson ratio ν_β. Finally, for both component types, the Rayleigh approximation of the damping matrix is employed: $\mathbf{B}_c = r_K \mathbf{K}_c + r_M \mathbf{M}_c$, with r_K and r_M being the Rayleigh stiffness and the Rayleigh mass, respectively.

2.3   Dynamic Simulation with Collisions

Initially at $t = 0$, all simulated cells are in a collision-free configuration. Each filopodium φ is associated to a root $\mathbf{r}_{\varphi\beta}$ which is located on the surface of the cell body β and initially, the distance $|\mathbf{r}_{\varphi\beta}, \mathbf{q}_{\varphi 0}| = 0$ where $\mathbf{q}_{\varphi 0}$ is the first node of the filopodium φ. For given cell body β, all the filopodium roots $\mathbf{r}_{\varphi\beta}$ are geometrically mapped to the mesh of parent body β: this mapping is implemented via barycentric coordinates of the root with respect to its embedding tetrahedron. The coordinates are computed at the initialization and remain constant during the simulation as described in [15]. Therefore, as the cell body moves, the filopodium roots strictly follow this motion.

Two sources of motions are applied to each cell: the center of each cell body is moved along a predefined trajectory, and the forces of predefined directions and amplitudes are applied to the filopodial tips. Then, given the actual configuration obtained in time t, the three phases of step $t + h$ consist in the following:

Unconstrained Dynamics. For each component c, (3) is assembled using the last known configuration given by $\mathbf{q}_c^t$ and $\dot{\mathbf{q}}_c^t$, and the corresponding system is solved with the constraint forces $\boldsymbol{\lambda} = 0$. The resulting velocity corrections $d\dot{\mathbf{q}}_c^{\text{uncon}}$ are integrated over the time step to get the unconstrained configuration given by the vector of positions $\mathbf{q}_c^{\text{uncon}}$ of each component of the simulated system. The assembled systems are solved directly, using a highly optimized solver based on the Thomas algorithm for block tridiagonal matrices [21] in the case of filopodia, and using the Pardiso solver [16] in the case of cell bodies. These solvers also construct the decomposition of the system matrix $\mathbf{A}_c$ needed to compute the Schur complement $\mathbf{H}_c \mathbf{A}_c^{-1} \mathbf{H}_c^\top$ later.

Collision Detection. During the unconstrained motion, individual cell bodies and their filopodia follow the Newton's law of physics as independent entities, which can possibly lead to the violations of equality and inequality constraints.

In the case of equality constraints, for each filopodium φ and its parent body β, the first node of the filopodium $\mathbf{q}_{\varphi 0}^{\text{uncon}}$ does not have to necessarily coincide with the current position of the corresponding filopodium root $\mathbf{r}_{\varphi\beta}^{\text{uncon}}$. Therefore, the violation is defined as the difference $\delta_E^{\text{uncon}} = |\mathbf{r}_{\varphi\beta}^{\text{uncon}} - \mathbf{q}_{\varphi 0}^{\text{uncon}}|$, with E running over all pairs of φ and β present in the simulation.

The violations of inequality constraints are computed by a proximity-based collision detection directly available in the SOFA framework [7]. It produces a vector of violations δ_I^{uncon}, with I running over all inter-penetrations between collision primitives associated to each filopodium and each cell body. The vector values correspond to the negative depths of individual inter-penetrations along the axis and surface normals for filopodia and cell bodies, respectively.

Besides the violations of both types of constraints, the corresponding rectangular matrices $\mathbf{H}_c$ are constructed for each component c, following the protocol introduced in [5]. In the case of equality constraints, the matrix contains the barycentric coordinates of the filopodium roots, and it maps the exact contact positions as they have occurred between particular collision primitives in the case of inequality constraints.

Collision Response. The vector of constraint forces $\boldsymbol{\lambda}$ (one force for each equality and inequality constraint) is to be found by solving (4). In the case of equality constraints, the constraint is satisfied if $\delta_E = 0$. In the case of inequality constraints representing frictionless contacts, the constraint is satisfied when it respects *Signorini's law* given as $\delta_I \leq 0 \perp \lambda_I \geq 0$, representing the complementarity of contact forces λ_I and positive gap δ_I between two objects. In other words, the inequality constraint is satisfied when either the negative violation becomes a positive gap (i.e., no contact occurs, so $\lambda_I = 0$) or non-zero contact forces are applied to remove the inter-penetration and then $\delta_I = 0$. The relation between the violations and correction forces is based on the Schur complement:

$$\delta_* = \delta_*^{\text{uncon}} + h[\mathbf{H}_c\mathbf{A}_c^{-1}\mathbf{H}_c^{\mathsf{T}} + \mathbf{H}_d\mathbf{A}_d^{-1}\mathbf{H}_d^{\mathsf{T}}]\boldsymbol{\lambda} \tag{4}$$

where c and d denote two components of the simulated system which are coupled by given constraint, and $*$ denotes either E or I subscripts. The c-d pair is always formed by one filopodium and one cell body for equality constraints, and any pair of colliding objects for inequality constraints.

Putting together the equations from all equality and inequality constraints, we arrive at a *linear complementarity problem*. We solve for $\boldsymbol{\lambda}$ using the projected Gauss-Seidel method [5]. Finally, the found vector of correction forces is used to perform the final set of corrections of each component, $\mathbf{q}_c^{t+h} = \mathbf{q}_c^{\text{uncon}} + \mathbf{A}_c^{-1}\mathbf{H}_c\boldsymbol{\lambda}$.

2.4   Generation of Cell Texture

Unlike the simulations limited to 2D image data, where the developers of simulation platforms have to cope with possibly overlapping cells, we model the cells fully in 3D space. These cells can touch one another, but they cannot mutually penetrate. Therefore, the texture of each cell is processed separately, following the protocol introduced in [18,19]. The texture of each simulated cell is represented as a cloud of many simulated fluorescent particles. They form a phantom image in which all cells are presented and in which the intensity of every voxel is proportional to the number of fluorescent particles that occupy the voxel volume. The initial distribution of these particles is taken from an image with an isotropic mosaic of procedural texture [13], being restricted to the cell volume. When rendering successive frames of the time-lapse sequence, the particle positions follow the cell geometry changes by tracking displacements of the specific mesh vertices. To obtain the final image that looks as if acquired using a fluorescence microscope, the phantom image is submitted to a virtual microscope [20]. In particular, the phantom image is blurred by an experimental point spread function of the real optical system, unevenly illuminated, resampled to the resolution of the simulated microscope setup, and finally degraded by photon shot noise, dark current, and read-out noise.

3   Results

To demonstrate the capability of our simulation system, we imitated the interactions of CRMP-2-overexpressing lung cancer cells, being transiently transfected with the green fluorescent protein conjugated to actin and exhibiting mesenchymal migration typical for cancer cell extravasation [9]. As a reference, we considered real 3D+t image data with the voxel size of $0.126 \times 0.126 \times 1.0 \,\mu m$, being acquired every two minutes using a spinning disk confocal microscope equipped with a water Plan-Apo $63 \times /1.20$ objective lens. The cells had variable cell body textures and protruded very short, single-branch filopodia of low motility.

We performed two simulations consisting of two and three mutually interacting motile cells, respectively, applying in each the time step of $h = 0.01 \,s$, Young's moduli of $E_\beta = 10 \,kPa$ and $E_\varphi = 500 \,kPa$, Poisson ratios of $\nu_\beta = 0.45$ and $\nu_\varphi = 0.4$, the Rayleigh mass and stiffness of 0.1 for both the cell bodies as well as filopodia, and the tolerance of 10^{-6} for the constraint solver used in (4). The shift of each cell body centroid over one time step was within $0.03 \,\mu m$, and the forces applied to the filopodial tips ranged from 100 to $200 \,\mu N$. The resulting 3D time-lapse sequences are shown in Fig. 1, demonstrating time-coherent, mechanics-based mutual interactions between the cell bodies, filopodia, and also between the cell bodies and the filopodia. In order to qualitatively compare the synthetic cell textures with its real counterparts, an example of four successive XY and XZ slices of both is depicted in Fig. 2. Their quantitative comparison was already given in [19], together with a more detailed description of the protocol that we followed here when generating the textures of multiple cells. The two complete synthetic sequences, accompanied by the inherently generated ground truth, and the source codes, developed to generate these two sequences, are made publicly available, free of charge for any research and noncommercial purposes, at http://cbia.fi.muni.cz/research/simulations/multiple-cells-filopodia.html.

In order to provide the reader with an estimate of how long the generation of the synthetic image data took, we measured the execution time of both simulations on a common workstation (Intel Xeon QuadCore 2.83 GHz, 32 GB RAM, Ubuntu 16.04 LTS). On average, the generation of one initial cell geometry took

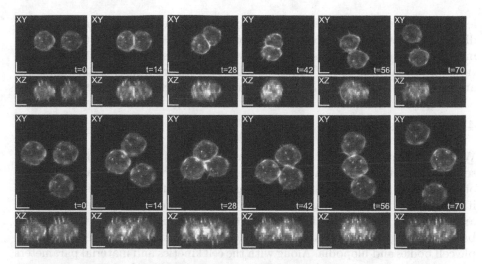

Fig. 1. Two maximum intensity projections of the resulting 3D+t sequences containing two (top) and three (bottom) interacting cells. The voxel size is $0.126 \times 0.126 \times 1.0\,\mu$m. The scale bars correspond to $5\,\mu$m.

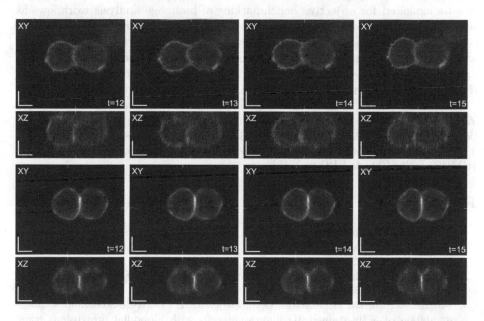

Fig. 2. An example of four successive XY and XZ slices of the real (top) and synthetic (bottom) image data of two colliding cells. The voxel size is $0.126 \times 0.126 \times 1.0\,\mu$m. The white ticks show the positions of the other two orthogonal cross-sections of image data. The scale bars correspond to $5\,\mu$m.

less than a minute. The modeling of cell motion and deformation, including handling of cell interactions, took roughly one and three minutes for the scenarios involving two and three cells, respectively. The image synthesis of 71 frames long time-lapse sequences of two and three cells, with the frame size of $336 \times 275 \times 18$ and $284 \times 375 \times 18$ voxels, respectively, took 56 and 84 min, respectively.

4   Conclusion

We have presented a simulation system that can generate synthetic 3D time-lapse sequences of multiple mutually interacting motile cells with filopodial protrusions of fixed geometries, accompanied by reference annotations. The system extends its predecessor [18,19], designed for single-cell, collision-unaware scenarios solely and proven to generate realistic cell textures, by adding proactive, mechanics-based handling of collisions to naturally deal with the interactions between multiple cell bodies and filopodia. Along with the cell kinetics and material parameters provided, the system allowed us to generate two plausible-looking synthetic 3D time-lapse sequences of multiple lung cancer cells with single-branch filopodia. Showing time-coherent, mechanics-constrained development, and being accompanied by inherently generated ground truth, such synthetic 3D+t image data can be exploited for objective benchmarking of bioimage analysis workflows as well as for training of deep-learning approaches that target fully 3D filopodium segmentation and tracking for multiple mutually interacting cells. In future work, we intend to extend our system with bleb-like protrusions and filopodia dynamically evolving their geometries over time, along with investigating an appropriate dynamic model for entire cell kinetics and its subsequent quantitative analysis.

Acknowledgments. This work was financially supported by the Czech Science Foundation [GJ16-03909Y to I.P., D.V.S., and M.M.], the Russian Science Foundation [17-11-01279 to D.V.S.], and the German Federal Ministry of Research and Education (BMBF) [031L0102 (de.NBI) to V.U.].

References

1. Barry, D.J., Durkin, C.H., Abella, J.V., Way, M.: Open source software for quantification of cell migration, protrusions, and fluorescence intensities. J. Cell Biol. **209**(1), 163–180 (2015)
2. Biswas, K.H., Zaidel-Bar, R.: Early events in the assembly of E-cadherin adhesions. Exp. Cell Res. **1**(358), 14–19 (2017)
3. Castilla, C., Maška, M., Sorokin, D.V., Meijering, E., Ortiz-de-Solorzano, C.: Segmentation of actin-stained 3D fluorescent cells with filopodial protrusions using convolutional neural networks. In: IEEE International Symposium on Biomedical Imaging, pp. 413–417 (2018)
4. Chenouard, N., et al.: Objective comparison of particle tracking methods. Nat. Methods **11**(3), 281–289 (2014)
5. Courtecuisse, H., Allard, J., Kerfriden, P., Bordas, S.P.A., Cotin, S., Duriez, C.: Real-time simulation of contact and cutting of heterogeneous soft-tissues. Med. Image Anal. **18**(2), 394–410 (2014)

6. Coutu, D.L., Schroeder, T.: Probing cellular processes by long-term live imaging-historic problems and current solutions. J. Cell Sci. **126**(17), 3805–3815 (2013)
7. Faure, F., et al.: SOFA: a multi-model framework for interactive physical simulation. In: Payan, Y. (ed.) Soft Tissue Biomechanical Modeling for Computer Assisted Surgery. SMTEB, vol. 11, pp. 283–321. Springer, Berlin (2012). https://doi.org/10.1007/8415_2012_125
8. Haeger, A., Wolf, K., Zegers, M.M., Friedl, P.: Collective cell migration: guidance principles and hierarchies. Trends Cell Biol. **25**(9), 556–566 (2015)
9. Jacquemet, G., Hamidi, H., Ivaska, J.: Filopodia in cell adhesion, 3D migration and cancer cell invasion. Curr. Opin. Cell Biol. **31**(10), 23–31 (2015)
10. Jacquemet, G., et al.: FiloQuant reveals increased filopodia density during breast cancer progression. J. Cell Biol. **216**(10), 3387–3403 (2017)
11. Nesme, M., Payan, Y., Faure, F.: Efficient, physically plausible finite elements. In: Eurographics, pp. 77–80 (2005)
12. Ortiz-de-Solórzano, C., Muñoz-Barrutia, A., Meijering, E., Kozubek, M.: Toward a morphodynamic model of the cell. Signal Process. Mag. **32**(1), 20–29 (2015)
13. Perlin, K.: An image synthesizer. In: SIGGRAPH, pp. 287–296 (1985)
14. Peterlík, I., et al.: Fast elastic registration of soft tissues under large deformations. Med. Image Anal. **45**(4), 24–40 (2018)
15. Peterlík, I., Duriez, C., Cotin, S.: Modeling and real-time simulation of a vascularized liver tissue. In: Ayache, N., Delingette, H., Golland, P., Mori, K. (eds.) MICCAI 2012. LNCS, vol. 7510, pp. 50–57. Springer, Heidelberg (2012). https://doi.org/10.1007/978-3-642-33415-3_7
16. Petra, C.G., Schenk, O., Lubin, M., Gärtner, K.: An augmented incomplete factorization approach for computing the Schur complement in stochastic optimization. SIAM J. Sci. Comput. **36**(2), C139–C162 (2014)
17. Przemieniecki, J.S.: Matrix structural analysis of substructures. Am. Inst. Aeronaut. Astronaut. J. **1**(1), 138–147 (1963)
18. Sorokin, D.V., Peterlík, I., Ulman, V., Svoboda, D., Maška, M.: Model-based generation of synthetic 3D time-lapse sequences of motile cells with growing filopodia. In: IEEE International Symposium on Biomedical Imaging, pp. 822–826 (2017)
19. Sorokin, D.V., et al.: FiloGen: a model-based generator of synthetic 3D time-lapse sequences of single motile cells with growing and branching filopodia. IEEE Trans. Med. Imaging (2018, in press). https://doi.org/10.1109/TMI.2018.2845884
20. Svoboda, D., Kozubek, M., Stejskal, S.: Generation of digital phantoms of cell nuclei and simulation of image formation in 3D image cytometry. Cytom. Part A **75A**(6), 494–509 (2009)
21. Thomas, L.H.: Elliptic problems in linear difference equations over a network. Watson Science Computer Lab Report, Columbia University, New York (1949)
22. Tsygankov, D., Bilancia, C.G., Vitriol, E.A., Hahn, K.M., Peifer, M., Elston, T.C.: CellGeo: a computational platform for the analysis of shape changes in cells with complex geometries. J. Cell Biol. **204**(3), 443–460 (2014)
23. Ulman, V., et al.: An objective comparison of cell-tracking algorithms. Nat. Methods **14**(12), 1141–1152 (2017)
24. Ulman, V., Svoboda, D., Nykter, M., Kozubek, M., Ruusuvuori, P.: Virtual cell imaging: a review on simulation methods employed in image cytometry. Cytom. Part A **89**(12), 1057–1072 (2016)
25. Urbančič, V., et al.: Filopodyan: an open-source pipeline for the analysis of filopodia. J. Cell Biol. **216**(10), 3405–3422 (2017)
26. Yao, Y., Smal, I., Meijering, E.: Deep neural networks for data association in particle tracking. In: IEEE International Symposium on Biomedical Imaging, pp. 458–461 (2018)

MRI to FDG-PET: Cross-Modal Synthesis Using 3D U-Net for Multi-modal Alzheimer's Classification

Apoorva Sikka[✉], Skand Vishwanath Peri, and Deepti R. Bathula

Indian Institute of Technology Ropar, Rupnagar, India
{apoorva.sikka,bathula}@iitrpr.ac.in
pvskand@gmail.com

Abstract. Recent studies suggest that combined analysis of Magnetic resonance imaging (MRI) that measures brain atrophy and positron emission tomography (PET) that quantifies hypo-metabolism provides improved accuracy in diagnosing Alzheimer's disease. However, such techniques are limited by the availability of corresponding scans of each modality. Current work focuses on a cross-modal approach to estimate FDG-PET scans for the given MR scans using a 3D U-Net architecture. The use of the complete MR image instead of a local patch based approach helps in capturing non-local and non-linear correlations between MRI and PET modalities. The quality of the estimated PET scans is measured using quantitative metrics such as MAE, PSNR and SSIM. The efficacy of the proposed method is evaluated in the context of Alzheimer's disease classification. The accuracy using only MRI is 70.18% while joint classification using synthesized PET and MRI is 74.43% with a p-value of 0.06. The significant improvement in diagnosis demonstrates the utility of the synthesized PET scans for multi-modal analysis.

1 Introduction

Alzheimer's disease (AD) is a chronic neuro-degenerative disorder that causes problems with memory, thinking and behavior. It is a progressive disease that gets worse with time, making early diagnosis very crucial [13]. Recently, various techniques using multi-modal image analysis have been proposed to identify bio-markers that aid in accurate diagnosis of AD [12]. It is evident that multiple modalities provide complementary information related to the disease, which when combined increases the efficacy of diagnosis. Joint analysis of positron emission tomography (PET) and magnetic resonance imaging (MRI) has been accepted as a method to diagnose AD [19]. While gray matter atrophy and ventricular enlargement in MRI are established markers for pathology, pattern of neuronal uptake and cerebral distribution of FDG in PET is also a discriminating factor for AD. However, PET in comparison to MRI is a relatively new modality and acquiring different modality scans for a single patient is not always feasible due to high cost, lack of imaging facilities and increased risk of radiation exposure. Current work attempts to use the information from MR image

© Springer Nature Switzerland AG 2018
A. Gooya et al. (Eds.): SASHIMI 2018, LNCS 11037, pp. 80–89, 2018.
https://doi.org/10.1007/978-3-030-00536-8_9

to estimate virtual PET scan and further explores the value of these synthetic PET scans in enhancing disease prediction accuracy when combined with MRI.

In recent years, various approaches based on machine learning have been proposed to predict one modality from another or a combination of other modalities. To reduce radiation dose [14], employs context-aware GANs to predict CT scans from MR scans. Similarly, a regression forest based framework was developed in [7] for predicting a standard-dose brain FDG-PET from a low-dose PET image and its corresponding MRI. A more challenging cross-modal synthesis task involves predicting functional scans from their corresponding structural scans. [10] used a patch based CNN which is capable of capturing non-linear mappings between PET and MRI. Few techniques based on partial least squares regression (PLSR) [12] or independent component analysis (ICA) [17], mapping non-local correlations have also been proposed.

There are two important aspects to consider when estimating FDG-PET images from their corresponding MRI Scans: (a) correlation between these modalities is not purely local or one-to-one; PET is a functional modality that quantifies hypo-metabolism and MR being a structural one measures brain atrophy [1,5] and (b) relationship between these modalities is quite complicated and nonlinear. The Fig. 1 shows corresponding slices of MR and PET scans of the same subject where the correlation values between local patches vary significantly in the range [−0.86, 0.94]. The technique in [10] based on deep learning uses patches that are defined in a local manner where a local patch of MR corresponds to a local patch of PET to learn the mapping. In contrast, the PLSR method [12] tries to capture global or non-overlapping correlations in the images, but maps inputs and outputs in a linear fashion. To effectively estimate PET from MR, the model has to capture relationships between non-adjacent voxels and learn non-linear mapping from MR to PET.

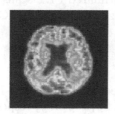 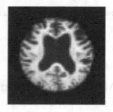

Fig. 1. A sample pair of MRI and its corresponding PET slice depict lack of one-to-one correspondence at individual voxels or local neighborhoods in terms of signal intensities and details.

Deep learning architectures have recently emerged as the most prominent and powerful techniques to learn complex non-linear transformations. Specifically, convolution neural networks (CNN) have been used to solve various problems like image recognition, segmentation and classification in computer vision. These models are hierarchical and have proved to be able to extract different types of features automatically. Unlike patch based networks that involve extracting and training using millions of patches (making them computationally inefficient), these networks directly process the entire input image to generate the final output image.

One such recently used network is deep convolutional auto-encoders based on U-Net architecture [15] with skip-like connections. In this work, conventionally unsupervised auto-encoders [18] are used in a supervised setting to learn a joint mapping between the two-modalities. But a major drawback for fully-connected networks is the increased chance of overfitting due to very large number of parameters and less training data available in medical images. Consequently, 3D fully convolutional network is employed that is not only capable of capturing global/non-local correlations but also models the input-output mapping using non-linear functions. The loss function used is binary cross-entropy as the loss function. As the accuracy of the predicted PET scans determines the success of any type of downstream analysis (classification, ROI analysis, etc.), the quality of the synthesized PET scans is thoroughly evaluated using quantitative metrics against ground truth. We have used three metrics namely, mean-absolute loss (MAE), peak signal-to-noise ratio (PSNR) and structural similarity index (SSIM). The efficacy of the proposed approach is further evaluated through multi-modal AD classification using logistic regression.

Our contributions in this paper are the following:

– We propose the first global and non-linear cross-modal approach for PET estimation from MR images via adapting 3D convolutional U-Net [2] architecture which takes care of non-local intensity correlations as well as non-linear mapping of input to output.
– We extensively evaluate our proposed cross-modal method against the existing patch based estimation method on three different metrics.
– We further assess the significance of estimated PET scans from the proposed method on the task of multi-modal Alzheimer's Disease Classification.

2   Methods

Given T1 weighted MRI scans represented as X and FDG-PET scans Y for k sample subjects with size $x_1 \times x_2 \times x_3$ and $y_1 \times y_2 \times y_3$ respectively. The task is to learn a mapping between the above mentioned modalities where every voxel in the given input scan is used to predict every voxel in the output scan. We use a 3D U-Net based architecture to estimate the corresponding PET scan. We have used gray matter (GM) from MRI scan as an input to the model. Gray Matter is used to estimate PET scan due to its high correlation in determining AD and normals. The architecture though is not a fully connected network but repetitive convolutions at multiple layers added with skip connections ensures that global correlations are captured.

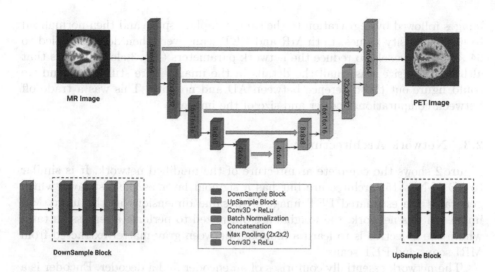

Fig. 2. 3D Regression U-Net architecture to generate a virtual PET scan using MRI scan.

2.1 Dataset

The experiments have been conducted on scans obtained from Alzheimer's Disease Neuroimaging Initiative (ADNI) database (adni.loni.usc.edu) [13]. A total of 384 subjects having both MRI and PET modalities (192 Normals and 192 AD) were used. We chose all the subjects that had both MR and PET images from the ADNI dataset available online. This includes scans from different populations from different areas as mentioned in [3]. Since we dont use any clinical score or demographic details as input or as ground truth in our method we did not mention details in the paper.

2.2 Preprocessing

As the downloaded ADNI dataset was not pre-processed, we implemented a manual pre-processing pipeline. MR Scans were first registered to MNI template space using FSL package [6].This was mandatory since all the images are of different sizes and registering them to a common space is required (to maintain homogeneity). All the images can be registered to a common image but we chose MNI since it is a standard template in the literature as mentioned in [9]. The registered scans were then skull-stripped using ROBEX [4] which were further normalized to [0–1] intensity values (to avoid the problem of gradients exploding and convergence). These preprocessed scans were then segmented into gray matter (GM), white matter (WM) and cerebral-spinal fluid (CSF) using FSL. There were multiple PET images for the same subject. So, we first registered all the other PET images to one of the reference PET and then we averaged all the registered PET images. These averaged out PET images were aligned to MR images followed by registration to the same template space and then normalized to [0–1] intensity values. Both MR and PET scans were then down sampled to $64 \times 64 \times 64$ voxels to reduce the network parameters (Fig. 3 clearly shows that although the size was small the details in the images were still intact and we could figure out the difference between AD and normals. This was a trade off between computational power and size of the image.)

2.3   Network Architecture

Figure 2 shows the complete architecture of the modified network. It is similar to 3D U-Net [15] architecture but has a sigmoid layer as the last layer which generates the estimated PET image with same dimensions as the input MR image. In this network, the weights are optimized to perform a regression task, where the objective is to learn a mapping between gray matter extracted from MRI scans and PET scans.

The network essentially comprises of an encoder and a decoder. Encoder is a modified convolutional network. It consists of $3 \times 3 \times 3$ convolutions followed by a rectified linear unit and a down-sampling operation performed using $2 \times 2 \times 2$ max pooling with a stride of 2. With each layer, we have increased the number of features maps. The decoder is an expanding network where every step consist of an upsampling followed by $3 \times 3 \times 3$ convolutions and batch normalization layers. In addition to the simple encoder-decoder architecture, there are skip connections which concatenate features of corresponding size from encoder to decoder layers. Although the inclusion of down-sampling layers leads to loss of information, the addition of skip connections between enocder and decoder helps retain some amount of information across higher layers from lower layers. This leads to generation of slightly smoother scans in comparison to ground truth. The final layer is $1 \times 1 \times 1$ convolution consisting of sigmoid activation which brings all values to [0–1] pixel range. Weights of the network are optimized in an end to end manner using binary cross entropy loss function as shown in equation:

$$H(y_t, \hat{y}_t) = - \sum_x y_t(x) \; log \; \hat{y}_t(x) \tag{1}$$

where where $\hat{y}_t$ is the predicted PET scan, y_t the ground truth PET scan and x is the total number of samples present in a batch.

3   Experiments

The proposed architecture was trained on NVIDIA Geforce GTX1080. For efficient use of the available data, 9-fold cross-validation was performed where 1 fold was used as a test set, 1 fold for validation and remaining 7 folds were used as training data. The learning rate was set to 0.008 and Adam [8] optimizer was used. The architecture is shown in Fig. 2 where number of feature maps of the model were chosen according to the GPU RAM. Total number of trainable parameters were 20M which is less as compared to a fully connected network and fully convolutional network [11] of similar size. U-Net introduces skip connections which enhances learning by merging various lower layer features to higher layers. The model was trained for 10 epochs.

The proposed method is evaluated against another comparative method by Li et al. [10] that models the relationship between MRI and PET in a local, nonlinear fashion. Firstly, preprocessed images were used to extract Gray Matter scans. Then, 3D patches from these images of size $15 \times 15 \times 15$ were extracted and the corresponding patch for the PET image of size $3 \times 3 \times 3$ is reconstructed. The method published in [10] was replicated to the maximum extent possible based on details provided in the paper, as the code is not available. All the parameters were kept as mentioned in the paper. The following section depicts the efficacy of the method by evaluating estimated PET scans both quantitatively and qualitatively. Quantitative evaluation is done using three different metrics based on correlation, perception and pixel intensities.

3.1 Mean Absolute Error (MAE)

MAE is a commonly used metric for any reconstruction problem. It gives us the average absolute difference between the estimated image and the ground truth intensity values. It is computed as follows:

$$MAE = \frac{\sum_{i=1}^{n} |y_i - x_i|}{n} \tag{2}$$

x_i and y_i are the intensity values of the pixels of estimated and actual PET.

3.2 Peak Signal-to-Noise Ratio (PSNR)

PSNR is mostly used as a quality measurement between two images. PSNR represents a measure of peak error. It is computed as follows:

$$PSNR = 10 \, log_{10} \left(\frac{MAX^2}{MSE} \right) \tag{3}$$

where MAX is the maximum possible intensity of the image and MSE is the mean squared error between the estimated and ground truth PET image.

3.3 Structure Similarity Index (SSIM)

Unlike MAE which measures the quality of an image based on pixel intensities, SSIM compares the similarity in structures of the two images. It is computed using the following equation:

$$SSIM(x, y) = \frac{(2\mu_x\mu_y + C_1) + (2\sigma_{xy} + C_2)}{(\mu_x^2 + \mu_y^2 + C_1)(\sigma_x^2 + \sigma_y^2 + C_2)} \tag{4}$$

where x is the estimated PET and y is the ground truth PET. μ_i is the mean of image i, σ_i is the variance of image i and σ_{xy} is the co-variance of images x

Table 1. Comparison of [10] with our proposed global approach for estimation of PET from MRI. For SSIM and PSNR metrics, the higher the value, better the estimation and for MAE metric, the lower the value, better the estimation.

Method	SSIM	MAE	PSNR
Li et al. [10]	0.5419 ± 0.044	0.0862 ± 0.0003	58.29 ± 1.337
Proposed method	$\mathbf{0.8211 \pm 0.015}$	$\mathbf{0.0422 \pm 0.006}$	$\mathbf{68.88 \pm 1.010}$

and y. C_1 and C_2 are empirically found constants in order to best perceive the structure of the estimated PET with respect to the ground truth.

Table 1 shows the performance of both the approaches using all three quantitative metrics. The high PSNR (68.88) and SSIM (0.82) and low MAE (0.0422) indicate that our proposed global method outperforms the local approach in all metrics, demonstrating the superiority of the architecture.

For a more qualitative analysis of the results, samples of PET scans estimated by both the approaches along with original PET scans are displayed in Fig. 3. The results clearly illustrate higher level of similarity between the PET scans estimated by the proposed method and their respective ground truth scans as compared to the alternative. The images further corroborate numerical results presented above and demonstrate the potential of the proposed approach to learn features corresponding to Normals and AD.

3.4 Impact of the Proposed Method on Alzheimer's Classification

To evaluate the effectiveness of the estimated PET scans, we performed classification of Alzheimer's Disease on the ADNI [13] dataset using reconstructed data. As 9 fold cross-validation was used as part of the cross-modality estimation procedure, the same setting was used to perform the classification task. To ensure consistency with [10], we used ℓ2-norm regularized logistic regression classifiers for both methods. The results of classification task using both the patch based method [10] and the proposed U-Net based method are shown in Table 2. As expected, we observe that the joint classification accuracy of MRI+Synthesized PET results in higher accuracy than stand alone MRI based classification due to the complementary nature of the features extracted and utilized from both modalities. The joint accuracy for [10] is less than that of only MRI might be due to considering only local correlations to generate the PET which is actually misclassifying the image. A paired sample t-test revealed marginally significant improvement ($p = 0.06$) in classification accuracy using MRI and synthesized PET images.

4 Discussion

We hypothesized that the correlation present between MRI and PET images is not local [12]. Ideally, a fully connected network (FCN) would be more appropriate to model global correlations between MRI and PET scans. However, due

Table 2. Accuracies on the binary classification task of AD vs Normal by the proposed method and the patch based method [10]. The second and the third columns (MRI & PET) have the same set of values as they are the classification accuracies on the original data and do not depend upon the method.

Method	MRI	PET	PET-Synthesis	MRI+PET-Synthesis
Li et al. [10]	70.18 ± 8.37	80.80 ± 7.95	60.33 ± 6.14	65.34 ± 5.43
Proposed method	70.18 ± 8.37	80.80 ± 7.95	**69.95 ± 5.59**	**74.43 ± 3.32**

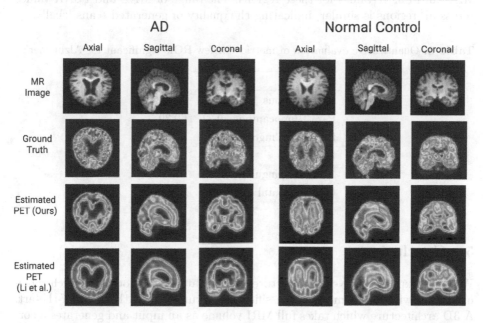

Fig. 3. Qualitative comparison of predicted PET scans with their corresponding true scans for 2 subjects – one from each group: Normal and AD in axial (right) and saggital views (left).

to large number of parameters and limited number of data samples, FCN produced relatively smoother estimates of PET scans. We initially experimented by training a supervised autoencoder architecture having two layers with each hidden layer having 500 and 300 hidden units. The number of parameters in this architecture in first layer itself rise to 131 million which increases the chances of overfitting given such less number of samples in medical images. With simple convolutional neural network the number of parameters reduces but the context it captures remains local. But U-Net is a convolutional encoder-decoder architecture with skip connections which helps us capture global correlations while keeping the number of parameters low.

We used binary crossentropy as loss function to train models instead of mean squared error (MSE) as it was generating jittery outputs, whereas the outputs were smooth in the former case. The choice of classifier was made to be consistent with [10], which could be improved by using deep learning based classifiers.

The estimated PET scans were evaluated against three global metrics as discussed above. Additionally, we tried to evaluate the quality of PET scans for few regions-of-interests (ROI) locally responsible for AD. For this, we parcellated estimated PET into 120 regions using AAL [16]. From these regions, we select few important regions highlighting AD as described in [5]. Table 3 highlights mean MAE and PSNR values for these regions. The range of MAE and PSNR values across all regions is similar, indicating the quality of generated scans locally.

Table 3. Quantitative evaluation of metrics for few ROIs significant for Alzhiemer's

Name	MAE	PSNR
Hippocampus	0.22	60.30
Para Hippocampus	0.22	60.39
Posterior Cingulate	0.21	60.58
Precuneus	0.18	61.52
Anterior Cingulate	0.16	61.14
Orbito Frontal	0.18	61.33

5 Conclusion

We have explored U-Net architecture to estimate PET modality which when used alongwith MRI improves classification accuracy over the state-of-the-art. A 3D architecture which takes full MRI volume as an input and generates a corresponding PET scan in one pass is used to perform the cross-modal estimation. The presence of skip connections allows the model to capture both non-linear and non-local correlations in an encoder-decoder setting. We have demonstrated the applicability of generated scans via performing multi-modality classification using both original MR and synthetic PET scan. The increased joint classification accuracies imply that synthetic data can be used in cases where capturing PET scans is not feasible. It can also be used as a missing data method for estimating PET scans that have been omitted for various reasons. We plan to extend this by making estimations more strong using adversarial training with the same U-Net architecture.

References

1. Ben-Cohen, A., et al.: Cross-modality synthesis from CT to PET using FCN and GAN networks for improved automated lesion detection. CoRR (2018)
2. Çiçek, Ö., Abdulkadir, A., Lienkamp, S.S., Brox, T., Ronneberger, O.: 3D U-Net: learning dense volumetric segmentation from sparse annotation. In: MICCAI (2016)

3. Demographics, A.: ADNI demographics (2012). adni.loni.usc.edu/wp-content/uploads/2012/08/ADNIEnrollDemographics.pdf
4. Iglesias, J.E., Liu, C.Y., Thompson, P.M., Tu, Z.: Robust brain extraction across datasets and comparison with publicly available methods. IEEE Trans. Med. Imaging **30**(9), 1617–1634 (2011)
5. Jack, C.R., et al.: Defining imaging biomarker cut points for brain aging and Alzheimer's disease. Alzheimer's Dement. **13**(3), 205–216 (2017)
6. Jenkinson, M., Beckmann, C.F., Behrens, T.E., Woolrich, M.W., Smith, S.M.: FSL. Neuroimage **23**, S208–S219 (2012)
7. Kang, J., et al.: Prediction of standard-dose brain PET image by using MRI and low-dose brain [18F] FDG PET images. Med. Phys. **49**(9), 5301–5309 (2015)
8. Kingma, D., Ba, J.: Adam: a method for stochastic optimization. In: International Conference on Learning Representations (2014)
9. Lakshmanan, A.G., Swarnambiga, A., Vasuki, S., Raja, A.A.: Affine based image registration applied to MRI brain. In: 2013 International Conference on Information Communication and Embedded Systems (ICICES) (2013)
10. Li, R., et al.: Deep learning based imaging data completion for improved brain disease diagnosis. In: Golland, P., Hata, N., Barillot, C., Hornegger, J., Howe, R. (eds.) MICCAI 2014. LNCS, vol. 8675, pp. 305–312. Springer, Cham (2014). https://doi.org/10.1007/978-3-319-10443-0_39
11. Long, J., Shelhamer, E., Darrell, T.: Fully convolutional networks for semantic segmentation. In: Proceedings of the IEEE Conference on Computer Vision and Pattern Recognition (2015)
12. Lorenzi, M., et al.: Multimodal image analysis in Alzheimers disease via statistical modelling of non-local intensity correlations. Scientific reports (2016)
13. Mueller, S.G., et al.: The Alzheimer's disease neuroimaging initiative. Neuroimaging Clin. N. Am. **15**(4), 869–877 (2005)
14. Nie, D., et al.: Medical image synthesis with context-aware generative adversarial networks. In: Descoteaux, M., Maier-Hein, L., Franz, A., Jannin, P., Collins, D.L., Duchesne, S. (eds.) MICCAI 2017. LNCS, vol. 10435, pp. 417–425. Springer, Cham (2017). https://doi.org/10.1007/978-3-319-66179-7_48
15. Ronneberger, O., Fischer, P., Brox, T.: U-net: convolutional networks for biomedical image segmentation. In: MICCAI 2015 (2015)
16. Tzourio-Mazoyer, N., et al.: Automated anatomical labeling of activations in SPM using a macroscopic anatomical parcellation of the MNI MRI single-subject brain. Neuroimage **15**(1), 273–289 (2002)
17. Vergara, V.M., Ulloa, A., Calhoun, V.D., Boutte, D., Chen, J., Liu, J.: A three-way parallel ICA approach to analyze links among genetics, brain structure and brain function. Neuroimage **98**, 386–394 (2014)
18. Vincent, P., Larochelle, H., Bengio, Y., Manzagol, P.A.: Extracting and composing robust features with denoising autoencoders. In: Proceedings of the 25th International Conference on Machine Learning, ICML 2008. ACM (2008)
19. Zhang, X.Y., Yang, Z.L., Lu, G.M., Yang, G.F., Zhang, L.J.: PET/MR imaging: new frontier in Alzheimer's disease and other dementias. Front. Mol. Neurosci. **10**, 343 (2017)

Tubular Network Formation Process Using 3D Cellular Potts Model

David Svoboda$^{(\boxtimes)}$, Tereza Nečasová, Lenka Tesařová, and Pavel Šimara

Centre for Biomedical Image Analysis, Masaryk University, Brno, Czech Republic
svoboda@fi.muni.cz

Abstract. The simulations in biomedical imaging serve when the real image data are difficult to be annotated or if they are of limited quantity. An increasing capability of contemporary computers allows to model and simulate complex shapes and dynamic processes. In this paper, we introduce a new model that describes the formation process of a complex tubular network of endothelial cells in 3D. This model adopts the fundamentals of cellular Potts model. The generated network of endothelial cells imitates the structure and behavior that can be observed in real microscopy images. The generated data may serve as a benchmark dataset for newly designed tracking algorithms. Last but not least, the observation of both real and synthetic time-lapse sequences may help the biologists to better understand and model the dynamic processes that occur in live cells.

Keywords: 3D cellular Potts model · Virtual cell
Volumetric image data · Network formation · Fractal dimension
Lacunarity

1 Introduction

The image based simulations focused on modeling of virtual cells and their behavior started to emerge in the early 90s. Before, they represented rather a theoretical approach which was understood to be an important one but not practically used. Nowadays, namely due to the increasing computational power, availability of multi-core processors or GPUs, and the capacity of contemporary computers, the development of new cell simulation frameworks goes hand in hand with newly emerging algorithms handling the biomedical image data. The current simulation frameworks can generate the synthetic image data accompanied with absolute ground truth in large quantities. The simulated data are either static [2,5] or dynamic [1,12].

The static data typically correspond to some images acquired with confocal or widefield fluorescence microscope. With this acquisition technique, only the subcellular components, that are under the scope, are fluorescently labeled and therefore visualized. This fact markedly simplifies the generated model of cell as there is no need to understand the whole cellular structure. On the other hand,

© Springer Nature Switzerland AG 2018
A. Gooya et al. (Eds.): SASHIMI 2018, LNCS 11037, pp. 90–99, 2018.
https://doi.org/10.1007/978-3-030-00536-8_10

the staining procedure, that precedes the acquisition of real images, takes some time. Moreover, in live cell imaging the staining may influence the behavior of the observed cells. For this purpose a phase contrast microscopy serves as an alternative solution and is very popular. This advantage is counterbalanced by the fact, that the synthetic model has to describe the whole cell structure and must be defined fully in 3D. The model, that would combine both or even multiple modalities (bright field microscopy [6], TIRF [8], or SMLM [9]) together, is a holy grail of simulations.

Even though there have been designed and implemented many simulation frameworks suitable for generation of time-lapse image sequence [15], most of them provided rather a schematic and simplified data. In [1], for example, the objects under the scope were the cells represented simply by touching or over-lapping spheres without any internal structure. In [12], the authors proposed a generator of a cell population. The cells were allowed to move and split due to mitosis. Nevertheless, the interaction between the cells was rather limited. In agent-based approach, the biologically motivated model is based on the modifica-tion [7] of standard cellular Potts model (CPM) [4] where the cells are expected to markedly interact. This approach was further extended [13] and the cells were allowed to be elongated as chords to resemble the behavior of real endothelial cells in tubular networks (see Fig. 1). The model was, however, settled in 2D only. This fact on one hand brings the advantage of high speed computation. On the other hand, the manipulation with 2D image data is very limiting, namely when simulating the behavior of phase contrast microscope, where the full 3D image information is required. In 2012, Scianna and Preziosi [10] designed a straightfor-ward extension of Merks' model into 3D. Later on, Svoboda and Kozubek [14] simplified Sianna's model and added the final post processing simulating the fluorescence as well as phase contrast microscope. Nevertheless, none of these two approaches offered a generation of straight elongated cells that occur in real images of tubular networks due to tension of the whole network. The tension forces caused some cells to be either unnaturally deformed or disjoint. In some particular cases some cells were even torn into pieces.

In this paper, we introduce a modification of previously mentioned CPM-based models. The newly presented model is defined fully in 3D space, keeps the already established mutual cell connections and guarantees the presence of chord-like cells that are exposed to tension forces. The synthetic image data produced by our approach are presented. A validation of similarity of both real and synthetic data using the fractal dimension and lacunarity descriptors is also provided.

2   Method

The proposed model combines the basic principles introduced in [10,14]. Let us first recall these principles. Afterwards, we emphasize the differences and introduce the new approach.

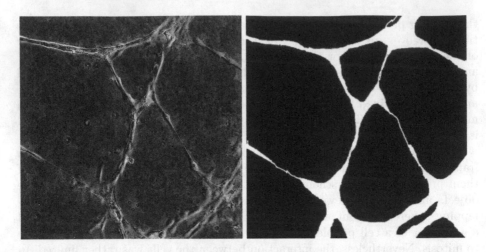

Fig. 1. An example of cell population forming a tubular network: (left) real image acquired using a phase-contrast microscope; (right) the left image annotated using two classes – foreground and background. Note, that all the images are volumetric ones. In order to visualize them we used maximum intensity projection.

2.1 3D Cellular Potts Model

Basic Definitions. Let $\Omega \subset \mathbb{R}^3$ be a three-dimensional lattice with each grid site $\mathbf{x} \in \Omega$ labeled with a spin function $\sigma \subset \Omega \times (\text{LABELS} \times \mathbb{N}_0 \times \mathbb{N}_0)$

$$\sigma : \mathbf{x} \rightarrow (label, id, cell). \tag{1}$$

where the individual elements have the meaning as follows:

- The property *label* defines the type of biological structure that the currently inspected grid site belongs to. The following set $\text{LABELS} = \{\text{nucleus},$ $\text{cytoplasm}, \text{mitochondrion}, \text{medium}, \text{ECM}\}$ is used. The first three labels correspond to subcellular components. The last two labels define the non-cellular objects appearing in the biological specimens. They are usually understood as a background. Here, ECM stands for *extra cellular matrix*.
- Inside each cell, there is just one nucleus. Nevertheless, some components appear twice or even multiple times. In order to distinguish between the individual occurrences of such objects a unique identifier $id \in \mathbb{N}_0$ is introduced. All the components are surrounded by the cytoplasm which is associated with one unique id.
- An element $cell \in \mathbb{N}_0$ is a unique identifier of a cell to which the currently inspected grid site $\mathbf{x}$ belongs.

In order to simplify the notation, let us define the name substitution $\sigma_{\text{bg}} = (bgLabel, 0, -)$, where $bgLabel \in \{\text{medium}, \text{ECM}\}$. The term σ_{bg} is therefore a value of spin function σ in a lattice site $\mathbf{x}$ that belongs to medium or ECM.

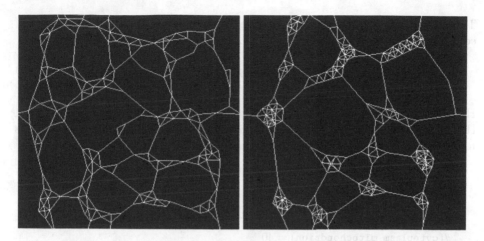

Fig. 2. An example of connectivity graph G: (left) shape of graph during the network evolution, (right) final configuration of the graph. Please note, that both graphs are defined fully in 3D. For visualization purposes a maximum intensity projection was used.

Finally, let $\pi_i, i \in \{1, 2, 3\}$ be a projection function that takes an element $\mathbf{x} = (x_1, x_2, x_3)$ of the Cartesian product $(X_1 \times X_2 \times X_3)$ to the value $\pi_i(\mathbf{x}) = x_i$. By using this projection, we can get, for example, the label of one particular grid site $\mathbf{x}$ by evaluating the term $\pi_1(\sigma(\mathbf{x}))$.

The 3D lattice Ω with its sites and spin function σ can be also understood as a discrete multichannel 3D image with individual voxels and voxel values. The voxels with similar values form the logical objects that we want to represent using the lattice Ω. In this case, the objects are the cells and their components.

Connectivity Preservation. In order to control the connectivity of neighboring cells, the graph based approach that tackles with the connectivity of CPM [13,14] is utilized. Here, a geometrical center of each cell is understood to be a vertex. The edge between two vertices is established if the corresponding cells touch using at least one voxel. This way, a non-oriented graph $G = (V, E)$ is constructed. Let $v \in V$ be any vertex in the graph G, then $d_G(v)$ is a number of all edges originating from v. In the very beginning, the graph G is disconnected, i.e., $\forall v \in V : d_G(v) = 0$. During the time, the nearby cells tend to join and the graph structure changes (see Fig. 2).

System Dynamics. The evolution of CPM is an iterative process that starts with an random initial distribution of cells rendered in the lattice Ω. One iteration of the CPM suggests to flip the spin function of a randomly selected grid site $\mathbf{x}_s$ (source) to a spin function $\sigma(\mathbf{x}_t)$ of its randomly selected neighbor $\mathbf{x}_t$ (target), and evaluates how this flip would affect the Hamiltonian H of the whole system:

$$\Delta H = \Delta H_{Adhesion} + \Delta H_{Shape} + \Delta H_{Chemotaxis}. \tag{2}$$

The term $H_{Adhesion}$ expresses the desire of individual grid site to either stay in contact with each other or to stay alone.

$$H_{Adhesion} = \sum_{\mathbf{x} \in \Omega, \mathbf{x}' \in N_{\mathbf{x}}} \left(1 - \delta_{\sigma(\mathbf{x}),\sigma(\mathbf{x}')}\right) J(\pi_1(\sigma(\mathbf{x})), \pi_1(\sigma(\mathbf{x}'))) \tag{3}$$

Here, $\delta_{x,y}$ is the Kronecker delta, $N_{\mathbf{x}}$ is a set of sites neighboring to $\mathbf{x}$. Finally, the $J \subset (\text{LABELS} \times \text{LABELS}) \times \mathbb{N}$ is a function that associates the binding penalties for individual pairs of components and is defined by an enumeration:

$J(\texttt{cytoplasm}, \texttt{ECM}) = 30$ $J(\texttt{medium}, \texttt{ECM}) = 0$
$J(\texttt{cytoplasm}, \texttt{medium}) = 40$ $J(\texttt{ECM}, \texttt{ECM}) = 0$
$J(\texttt{cytoplasm}, \texttt{cytoplasm}) = 10$ $J(\texttt{medium}, \texttt{medium}) = 0$
$J(\texttt{cytoplasm}, \texttt{nucleus}) = 40$ $J(other, other) = 10000$
$J(\texttt{cytoplasm}, \texttt{mitochondrion}) = 40$

The term H_{Shape} imposes geometrical constrains. In this case, the cell volume (number of grid sites per cell) constraint is employed:

$$H_{Shape} = \lambda_{volume} \sum_{L,C} (vol_{L,C} - Vol_L)^2 \tag{4}$$

where λ_{volume} is a weight defining the influence of this term, C is an cell id, L is a cell component id, $vol_{L,C}$ is the current volume of a component L in cell C, and Vol_L is an mean expected volume of components with label L.

The term $\Delta H_{Adhesion}$ (ΔH_{Shape}) expresses the difference between $H_{Adhesion}$ (H_{Shape}) calculated with the new suggested value of $\sigma(\mathbf{x}_t)$ and $H_{Adhesion}$ (H_{Shape}) with the original value $\sigma(x_s)$.

Finally, the term $\Delta H_{Chemotaxis}$ expresses the cell ability to respond to the chemical stimulus. Each cell detects the concentration of signals (the biological material which is produced by each cell and which serves as an attractor to other cells) in its vicinity and tries to occupy the position with the highest positive gradient of concentration $c(\cdot, \cdot)$. The term is expressed as:

$$\Delta H_{Chemotaxis} = -\left(1 - \delta_{\sigma(\mathbf{x}_s),\sigma_{\text{bg}}}\right) \lambda_{chemical} \left[c(\mathbf{x}_t, t) - c(\mathbf{x}_s, t)\right] \tag{5}$$

where $\lambda_{chemical}$ is a parameter controlling the importance of cell chemotaxis and $c(\mathbf{x}, t)$ is the current (time t) concentration of the signals at the site $\mathbf{x}$. The term $c(\mathbf{x}_t, t) - c(\mathbf{x}_s, t)$ defines the difference in concentrations between the current $\mathbf{x}_s$ and the proposed $\mathbf{x}_t$ sites. The concentration function $c(\cdot, \cdot)$ is defined by the following equation (arguments were dropped):

$$\frac{\partial c}{\partial t} = D\nabla^2 c + \beta(\mathbf{x}, t)(1 - \delta_{\sigma(\mathbf{x}),\sigma_{\text{bg}}}) - \frac{1}{\gamma}\delta_{\sigma(\mathbf{x}),\sigma_{\text{bg}}} c \tag{6}$$

where $\beta(\mathbf{x}, t)$ is the secretion rate of the signals released from the cell that occupies the site $\mathbf{x}$, γ is the half life of signals in the medium, and D is the diffusion coefficient. The secretion rate β is a decreasing function, i.e., if given cell acquires sufficient number of attachments with surrounding cells, it decreases the production of signals c:

$$\beta(\mathbf{x}, t) = \begin{cases} \alpha \cdot 0.9995^{(t-t_0)} & \text{if} \quad d_G(\pi_3(\sigma(\mathbf{x}))) \geq 2 \\ \alpha & \text{otherwise} \end{cases} \qquad (7)$$

Here, α is a initial secretion rate identical for all the cells, and t_0 is the time when the given cell $\pi_3(\sigma(\mathbf{x}))$ first attached at least two other cells.

The probability of flipping the spin of the lattice site $\mathbf{x}_s$ to the spin $\sigma(\mathbf{x}_t)$ is then given as:

$$P(\sigma(\mathbf{x}_t) \leftarrow \sigma(\mathbf{x}_s)) = \begin{cases} e^{-\Delta H/T} & \text{if } \Delta H > 0, \\ 1 & \text{if } \Delta H \leq 0. \end{cases} \qquad (8)$$

where T is a temperature describing the willingness of cells to move.

2.2   The Proposed Modifications

Intra-Cell Compactness. In [7], Merks et al. introduced a method that kept each cell to be compact. The algorithm took the pixel, which value was proposed to be changed, and compared it with the values of its neighbors. The check for the local compactness was based on the inspection of individual neighbors in the clock-wise manner. Unfortunately, this approach could not be straightforwardly extended to 3D space. For this purpose, we propose a new method which works well for 3D and can be extended to any higher dimension. The procedure checks if the proposed change of the value in the inspected voxel would keep or violate the compactness of the cell to which this voxel belongs. The procedure is as follows:

1. Let $\mathbf{x} \in \Omega$ be an inspected voxel belonging to some cell and let $N_{\mathbf{x}}$ be its $3 \times 3 \times 3$ neighborhood.
2. Collect the labels from grid Ω in the neighbourhood $N_{\mathbf{x}}$, keep their positions, and create a 3D labeled image K as follows: $\forall \mathbf{p} \in N_{\mathbf{x}} : K(\mathbf{p} - \mathbf{x}) = \pi_1(\sigma(\mathbf{p}))$.
3. Count, how many voxels in K belong to background (`medium` or `ECM`) and store the result as value a.
4. Count, how many different labels are included in K and store the result as value b.
5. Derive a binary image K_b from K by setting voxels with the same label, as the central voxel has, to *true*.
6. Set the central voxel value in K_b to *false* to simulate the proposed voxel value change.
7. Find any voxel with value *true* in K_b and run the flood-fill algorithm starting from this voxel. The filling value is *false*.
8. Try to find again any voxel with value *true* in K_b.
9. If the last search was successful and $(a > 0$ or $b \geq 2))$ then mark the proposed voxel value change in $\mathbf{x}$ as undesirable as this change would split the cell into at least two pieces.

Tension Forces. The tension and stress inside the network is strongly influenced by the chemotactic term (5). In the following text, we propose a modification of this term and, afterwards, check how it influences the formation of network structure in 3D space.

As soon as some cell detects a remarkable drop of signal concentration c in its vicinity, it starts to starve. We propose this cell to stop using the term $\Delta H_{Chemotaxis}$ and also all the cells reachable from this cell through the graph G change their behavior analogously.

Due to the proposed change, the term $\Delta H_{Adhesion}$ becomes more dominant. Together with the shape term ΔH_{Shape} it keeps the volume of each cell at a given mean value and pushes each cell to have the lowest possible surface. This constraint applied to two neighboring connected cells, that are pulled from each other, produces elongated and smoothly thinning connection. This is, however, not the case of 3D model, where the lowest possible surface requires the cells to look like ideal spheres, while connections are formed of unnaturally twisted one voxel wide curves. The difference stems from the fact, that 2D model is a just a cross section of the 3D model and does not properly describe the real organization of cells in 3D space. In order to get smoothly thinning and strain connection between each two connected cells in 3D model, we propose the following modification of each CPM iteration:

1. Take a current graph G and render it into the image of the same size as the lattice Ω is (see an example in Fig. 2).
2. Compute the 3D Euclidean distance map (EDM) over this image.
3. If a grid site $\mathbf{x}$, that belongs to some cell, is proposed to become a background grid site (`medium` or `ECM`) and the EDM($\mathbf{x}$) $< width$, where $width$ is a minimum acceptable width of the connection between the cells, we reject this change proposal.

3   Results and Validation

The objective of this paper was to propose a model that describes the structure of the tubular network and its evolution in the course of time. From the biological point of view, the most important aspect is the final configuration of the network. The biologists inspect the structure of the network and the organization of the cells. For this reason, we focus our interest on the generated images that record the network in a stable configuration, i.e., when it stops evolving. In Fig. 3, you can see a sample final network as a rendered volumetric image. As it is difficult to imagine the exact shape of the network in the perspective projection, we also offer a maximum intensity projection of this particular network in Fig. 4 (bottom-left image). In the given figure, you can also inspect other synthetically generated networks (bottom row) and visually compare them with the real networks (upper row), that were obtained by manual annotation of real microscopy images.

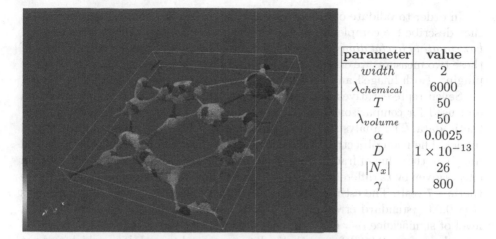

parameter	value
$width$	2
$\lambda_{chemical}$	6000
T	50
λ_{volume}	50
α	0.0025
D	1×10^{-13}
$|N_x|$	26
γ	800

Fig. 3. 3D visualization of synthetic tubular network using Paraview software together with a list of parameters that were used for the creation of this artificial network.

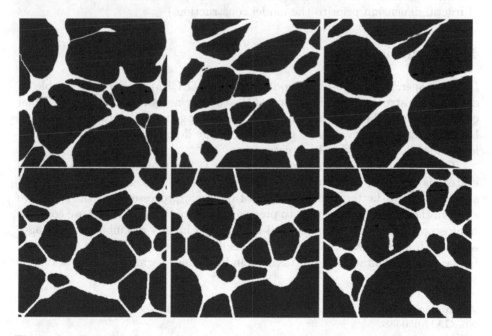

Fig. 4. A collection of images representing the mask of tubular network of endothelial cells. The first row contains the real images, the second one the synthetic ones. For the visualization purposes, the maximum intensity projection is utilized.

In order to validate our model, we decided to employ the standard measures that describe the complexity of the structures depicted in the analyzed images: *box counting fractal dimension* and *lacunarity* [3, 11]. As a tool for computation of these two measures we employed the *ImageJ* software[1] together with the *FracLac* plugin[2]. Both ImageJ and FracLac are freely available.

Seven representatives from real data were randomly selected for annotation and used for comparison to seven randomly selected representatives from synthetic data. The analysis of these images was performed using a linear mixed model. The main objective was to inspect the effect of being a synthetic or real image on the value of fractal dimension or lacunarity with respect to the random effects given by 12 different measurements for each of 14 individual images (7 synthetic + 7 real). The estimated effect of synthetic data on fractal dimension was $\beta = 0.031$ (standard error: 0.018), which was not significant (p-value = 0.137, level of significance $\alpha = 0.05$). In case of lacunarity the change was $\beta = -0.068$ (standard error: 0.096) for synthetic data compared to real data, which was not significant (p-value = 0.666, level of significance $\alpha = 0.05$). Thus, there were no significant differences between the real and synthetic data in terms of fractal dimension and lacunarity. (The logarithm transformation was used for the values of fractal dimension prior to the model construction.)

4 Conclusions

In this paper, we proposed a modification of 3D CPM model that is able to describe the structure and evolution of the tubular network of living endothelial cells. In order to check the plausibility of computer generated data, we submitted both real and synthetic images to selected image descriptors and showed a high level of similarity between both categories.

The proposed model (the implementation is freely available[3]) and the generated data can be used for the verification of some biological hypothesis and subsequently to better understanding of dynamic processes that occur in live cells. In the future, we also plan to properly simulate the optics of phase contrast microscope to be able to create real-like looking images resembling the images acquired from the real microscope. In this sense, we would be able to produce image datasets suitable for the tasks including image segmentation, tracking or reconstruction.

Acknowledgments. This work was supported by Czech Science Foundation, grant No. GA17-05048S.

---

[1] https://imagej.net/.

[2] https://imagej.nih.gov/ij/plugins/fraclac/fraclac.html.

[3] https://cbia.fi.muni.cz/research/simulations/multicomponent-cpm.html.

References

1. Dufour, A., Thibeaux, R., Labruyère, E., Guillén, N., Olivo-Marin, J.C.: 3-D active meshes: fast discrete deformable models for cell tracking in 3-D time-lapse microscopy. IEEE Trans. Image Process. **20**(7), 1925–1937 (2011)
2. Ghaye, J., Micheli, G., Carrara, S.: Simulated biological cells for receptor counting in fluorescence imaging. BioNanoScience **2**, 94–103 (2012)
3. Gould, D.J., Vadakkan, T.J., Poché, R.A., Dickinson, M.E.: Multifractal and lacunarity analysis of microvascular morphology and remodeling. Microcirculation **18**, 136–151 (2011)
4. Graner, F., Glazier, J.A.: Simulation of biological cell sorting using a two-dimensional extended Potts model. Phys. Rev. Lett. **69**(13), 2013–2016 (1992)
5. Lehmussola, A., Ruusuvuori, P., Selinummi, J., Huttunen, H., Yli-Harja, O.: Computational framework for simulating fluorescence microscope images with cell populations. IEEE TMI **26**(7), 1010–1016 (2007)
6. Malm, P., Brun, A., Bengtsson, E.: Papsynth: simulated bright-field images of cervical smears. In: International Symposium on Biomedical Imaging: From Nano to Macro, pp. 117–120. IEEE Press (2010)
7. Merks, R.M., Brodsky, S.V., Goligorksy, M.S., Newman, S.A., Glazier, J.A.: Cell elongation is key to in silico replication of in vitro vasculogenesis and subsequent remodeling. Dev. Biol. **289**(1), 44–54 (2006)
8. Rezatofighi, S.H., et al.: A framework for generating realistic synthetic sequences of total internal reflection fluorescence microscopy images. In: International Symposium on Biomedical Imaging, pp. 157–160 (2013)
9. Sage, D., et al.: Quantitative evaluation of software packages for single-molecule localization microscopy. Nat. Methods-Tech. Life Sci. Chem. **12**(8), 717–724 (2015)
10. Scianna, M., Preziosi, L.: Multiscale developments of the cellular Potts model. Multiscale Model. Simul. **10**(2), 342 (2012)
11. Smith, T., Lange, G., Marks, W.: Fractal methods and results in cellular morphology - dimensions, lacunarity and multifractals. J. Neurosci. Methods **69**(2), 123–136 (1996)
12. Svoboda, D., Ulman, V.: MitoGen: a framework for generating 3D synthetic time-lapse sequences of cell populations in fluorescence microscopy. IEEE Trans. Med. Imaging **36**(1), 310–321 (2017)
13. Svoboda, D., et al.: Vascular network formation in silico using the extended cellular Potts model. In: IEEE International Conference on Image Processing, pp. 3180–3183, September 2016
14. Svoboda, D., Kozubek, M.: Multimodal simulations in live cell imaging. In: Tsaftaris, S.A., Gooya, A., Frangi, A.F., Prince, J.L. (eds.) SASHIMI 2017. LNCS, vol. 10557, pp. 89–98. Springer, Cham (2017). https://doi.org/10.1007/978-3-319-68127-6_10
15. Ulman, V., Svoboda, D., Nykter, M., Kozubek, M., Ruusuvuori, P.: Virtual cell imaging: a review on simulation methods employed in image cytometry. Cytom. Part A **89**(12), 1057–1072 (2016)

Deep Learning Based Coronary Artery Motion Artifact Compensation Using Style-Transfer Synthesis in CT Images

Sunghee Jung[1], Soochahn Lee[2]([✉]), Byunghwan Jeon[1], Yeonggul Jang[1], and Hyuk-Jae Chang[3]

[1] Brain Korea 21 PLUS Project for Medical Science, Yonsei University, Seoul 03722, South Korea
sh.jung@yonsei.ac.kr
[2] Department of Electronic Engineering, Soonchunhyang University, Asan 31538, South Korea
sclsch@sch.ac.kr
[3] Division of Cardiology, Severance Cardiovascular Hospital, Yonsei University College of Medicine, Yonsei University Health System, Seoul 03721, South Korea

Abstract. Motion artifact compensation of the coronary artery in computed tomography (CT) is required to quantify the risk of coronary artery disease more accurately. We present a novel method based on deep learning for motion artifact compensation in coronary CT angiography (CCTA). The ground-truth, i.e., coronary artery without motion, was synthesized using full-phase four-dimensional (4D) CT by applying style-transfer method because it is medically impossible to obtain in practice. The network for motion artifact compensation based on very deep convolutional neural network (CNN) is trained using the synthesized ground-truth. An observer study was performed for the evaluation of the proposed method. The motion artifacts were markedly reduced and boundaries of the coronary artery were much sharper than before applying the proposed method, with a strong inter-observer agreement (kappa = 0.78).

Keywords: Motion artifact compensation · Coronary artery
Deep learning · Computed tomography · Style-transfer

1 Introduction

Coronary artery disease (CAD), also known as ischemic heart disease, is the leading cause of death globally [7]. Recently, non-invasive coronary computed tomography angiography (CCTA) has been widely adopted. If CCTA is acquired when the heart is beating, motion artifacts can inevitably be caused. Therefore, motion artifact compensation is required to quantify the severity of CAD more accurately.

© Springer Nature Switzerland AG 2018
A. Gooya et al. (Eds.): SASHIMI 2018, LNCS 11037, pp. 100–110, 2018.
https://doi.org/10.1007/978-3-030-00536-8_11

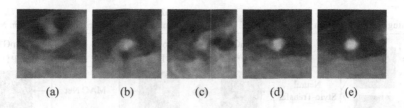

(a)   (b)   (c)   (d)   (e)

Fig. 1. Appearance of the motion artifacts of a coronary artery in different phases of same patient's 4D CT according to a 5-point Likert scale, described in Sect. 3.2 (a) completely unreadable, (b) significant motion artifacts, (c) apparent motion artifacts, (d) minor motion artifacts, (e) no motion artifacts

To solve this problem, prospective ECG-gating or drugs (e.g., beta-blockers) can be used. The former enables data acquisition when the heart is moving as quiescently as possible, and the latter enables the patient heart rate to be reduced. Nonetheless, motion artifacts can occur if the heart rate is irregular or due to the temporal resolution of CT.

Various approaches based on image processing have been proposed to solve this issue. Several methods were proposed that first perform coronary artery motion estimation, after which the cardiac CT images are obtained using motion compensated reconstruction [1,9,14,16]. However, the motion artifacts are likely to degrade the performance of motion estimation, ultimately leading to the degradation of motion compensation as well.

The advancement of deep learning has caused revolutionary improvements across many different disciplines [3,8,13]. It is reasonable to assume that a physician could estimate the image without the motion artifacts more accurately with more experience. Based on this assumption, together with the success of deep learning methods, we hypothesized that deep learning can be used for motion artifact compensation as well.

In this work, we approach the issue of reducing motion artifacts in CCTA by using deep learning, similar to denoising [17] or super-resolution methods [11] that have recently been shown successful. To apply deep learning to coronary artery motion compensation, ground-truth (GT) data are required. However, the image of a coronary artery without motion in a patient cannot be determined. That is, it is medically impossible to obtain exactly the corresponding coronary CT images with and without motion artifacts.

Our core idea is to use a style transfer method on the image patches from four-dimensional (4D) CT images, containing phases with large and small amounts of motion artifacts (Fig. 1), to generate a synthetic ground truth, which we term SynGT. We apply style transfer, instead of just using only the patches directly, owing to the local deformations that occur from the heartbeats. Our aim is to suppress the effect of genuine appearance change and isolate only the effect of motion artifacts. Using the SynGT, we can subsequently learn to generate images with reduced motion artifacts from the corresponding training input images.

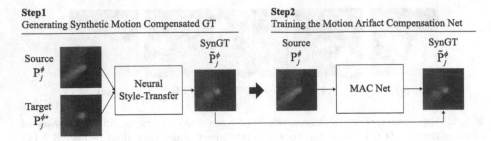

Fig. 2. Workflow of the proposed method. In step 1, generate synthetic motion compensated patch (SynGT) using style-transfer method. In step 2, training the motion artifact compensation network (MAC Net) using SynGT. The detailed descriptions of step 1 and step 2 are found in Sects. 2.2 and 2.3, respectively.

The primary contributions of our work are summarized as follows, (i) we applied the style transfer method in order to synthesize the motion compensated ground truth (SynGT) (Step1 in Fig. 2), (ii) trained the motion artifact compensation network, which we termed MAC Net, by utilizing the SynGT (Step2 in Fig. 2), and (iii) performed an observer study that scores the degree of motion artifacts before and after applying the proposed method.

Section 2 examines the proposed method and the details are presented in each subsection. Section 3 shows the dataset and experimental results of the proposed method. In Sect. 4, we present the conclusions and discussions.

2   Methods

2.1   Extraction of Corresponding Coronary Patches from 4D CT

We used 4D CT images which are acquired by retrospective gating using a dual source CT scanner (SOMATOM Definition Flash, Siemens). All raw data were reconstructed 0%–90% in 10% increments of the R-R interval.

Herein, we specifically focus only on the middle of the right coronary artery (mid-RCA), which generally has the most motion, as the region of interest when we trained the motion artifact compensation (MAC) network. Given the temporally sampled three-dimensional (3D) CT volumes, the mid-RCA was manually annotated by the experts in each volume using a commercial coronary analysis software (QAngioCT, Medis Medical Imaging Systems, Leiden, Netherlands). Here, the 1st right ventricle branch and acute marginal branch are defined as the start point and the end point, respectively.

The mid-RCA centerline $\mathcal{C}^\phi$ of a 3D volume at phase ϕ is represented as a discretized set of ordered 3D coordinates $\mathcal{C}^\phi = \left\{ c_i^\phi | 0 \leq i \leq N_c^\phi - 1 \right\}$, where c_i^ϕ denotes the i_{th} 3D point coordinate, among a total number of N_c^ϕ, of $\mathcal{C}^\phi$. The exact centerline is approximated as a piecewise linear function between the points in $\mathcal{C}^\phi$. Thus, the entire length of the mid-RCA centerline is defined

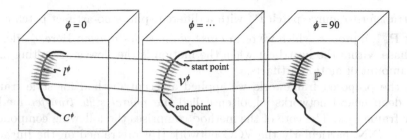

Fig. 3. Determining positions and normals for corresponding patches of mid-RCA in 3D CT volumes at different temporal phases, included within the full-phase 4D CT volumes. The centerlines of the mid-RCA, including the start and end points are manually annotated in full-phase volumes.

as the sum of all distances between subsequent point pairs, and denoted as $l^\phi = \sum_{i=0}^{i<N-1} ||c_{i+1}^\phi - c_i^\phi||_2$.

To extract the corresponding patches on $\mathcal{C}^\phi$, the corresponding points must first be determined. We assume that the start and end points for all ϕ will correspond because they correspond to the same anatomical landmark. A fixed number of M equidistant points $\mathcal{V}^\phi = \left\{ q_j^\phi | 0 \leq j \leq M - 1 \right\}$ each spaced $\frac{l^\phi}{M}$ are sampled between the start and end points of $\mathcal{C}^\phi$. Because the mid-RCA centerline is approximated as a piecewise linear function, we applied interpolation to compute the exact equidistant point coordinate. Finally, we define the normal directions n_j^ϕ for the planar patches centered at each q_j^ϕ as the tangential direction of $\mathcal{C}^\phi$ at q_j^ϕ. Figure 3 visualizes this process of determining the corresponding points along 3D CT volumes at different temporal phases.

The corresponding patches $\mathbb{P} = \left\{ \mathbf{P}_j^\phi | 0 \leq j \leq M - 1 \right\}$ are extracted by sampling the voxel intensities on an $R \times R$ discrete grid centered at q_i^ϕ with normal n_j^ϕ within the corresponding 3D CT volume. To align the spatial distribution of the grid points physically, we constructed a two-dimensional grid (on the xy-plane as reference) with 3D coordinates considering the physical dimensions of the CT, and applied translation based on the center point, and rotation based on the normal direction to obtain the projected grid coordinates. Because these coordinates are not integers, bicubic interpolation is applied when assigning intensity values to each pixel in the extracted patch.

2.2 Generating Synthetic Motion Compensated Patches Using Cross-Phase Style-Transfer

The motion of the heartbeat causes differences in its local appearance. However, we would like to obtain the corresponding patch with the identical local appearance but without motion artifacts because we would like to train a convolutional neural network (CNN) to remove only the artifacts. As this is clinically unattainable, we aim to synthesize this same-phase-no-artifact patch, $\tilde{\mathbf{P}}_j^\phi$, using style transfer to source patch $\mathbf{P}_j^\phi$ with a different-phase-no-artifact patch as the target $\mathbf{P}_j^{\phi\star}$, a process which we term *cross-phase style-transfer*. Here, $\phi\star$ denotes the phase within the heartbeat when the motion is the slowest, resulting in the least amount of motion artifacts.

In the proposed framework, we applied a recent method for style transfer using deep neural networks [5], often called the *neural style transfer* method, in our framework. The core of the method comprises the following components. First, a CNN, particularly the VGG network [15] pretrained on the ImageNet database [4], is used to compute local image features that are subsequently defined as the numerical representation of the content. If we denote the tensor of the CNN features at layer l as $\mathbf{F}_x^l$ and $\mathbf{F}_c^l$ for the synthesized image $\boldsymbol{I_x}$ and content reference image $\boldsymbol{I_c}$, respectively, the loss function for the content is defined as

$$\mathcal{L}_{content}\left(\boldsymbol{I_x}, \boldsymbol{I_c}\right) = \frac{1}{2}\|\boldsymbol{I_x} - \boldsymbol{I_c}\|_2^2. \tag{1}$$

Next, the numerical representation of the style is defined using the Gram matrix $\mathbf{G}^l$, where each element is the inner product between different CNN features at layer l, as

$$G_{ij}^l = \mathbf{F}_i^l \cdot \mathbf{F}_j^l, \tag{2}$$

where G_{ij}^l denotes the element at row i, column j of $\mathbf{G}^l$. $\mathbf{F}_i^l$ and $\mathbf{F}_j^l$ denote the i_{th} and j_{th} features, respectively corresponding to the i_{th} and j_{th} convolutional kernels, respectively, at layer l. The loss function for style is subsequently defined as

$$\mathcal{L}_{style}\left(\boldsymbol{I_x}, \boldsymbol{I_s}\right) = \frac{1}{2N_x^{l^2} \times 2N_s^{l^2}}\|\mathbf{G}_x^l - \mathbf{G}_s^l\|_2^2, \tag{3}$$

where G_x^l and G_s^l are the Gram matrices, and N_x^l and N_s^l are the number of features at layer l, for $\boldsymbol{I_x}$ and style-reference image $\boldsymbol{I_s}$, respectively. Finally, $\boldsymbol{I_x}$ is determined by using a gradient descent to minimize the balanced loss, defined as

$$\mathcal{L}_{total}\left(\boldsymbol{I_x}, \boldsymbol{I_c}, \boldsymbol{I_s}\right) = \alpha\mathcal{L}_{content}\left(\boldsymbol{I_x}, \boldsymbol{I_c}\right) + \beta\mathcal{L}_{style}\left(\boldsymbol{I_x}, \boldsymbol{I_s}\right), \tag{4}$$

where α and β are coefficients to balance the effect between the content and style loss terms. We note that CNN is just applied as a tool to compute the features, and that optimization of Eq. 4 is for modifying the input image so that its style resembles that of the target image, not for learning parameters of the CNN.

From the review above, $\tilde{\mathbf{P}}_j^\phi$, $\mathbf{P}_j^\phi$, and $\mathbf{P}_j^{\phi\star}$ correspond to $\boldsymbol{I_x}$, $\boldsymbol{I_c}$, and $\boldsymbol{I_s}$, respectively. While the phase $\phi\star$ with the least amount of motion is determined manually, the patches from all other phases ϕ can be assigned as the source, i.e., the reference patch for content $\mathbf{P}_j^\phi$.

2.3   Training and Applying the Motion Artifact Compensation Network

We adopted the very deep CNN for super-resolution (VDSR) network [11], originally applied to super-resolution, in our problem of motion artifact compensation. We chose VDSR because (1) our problem is primarily a noise reduction

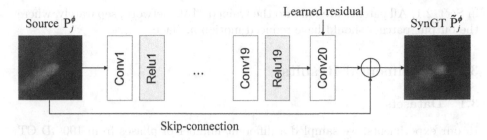

Fig. 4. Architecture of the MAC network, based on the VDSR network [11]. A pair of convolutional layers and an activation function are cascaded repeatedly. The last convolutional layer denotes a learned residual image. A single skip-connection from the input to output is applied.

problem, and noise reduction is similar to achieving super-resolution, (2) the input is upsampled such that patch sizes of the input and output are assumed to be the same for the VDSR as our configuration, and (3) it shows good performance and fast convergence during training.

The good performance is primarily due to the deep structure of the network, which combines the very deep CNN model of [15] together with the residual learning of [6]. Meanwhile skip connections were added at every other convolutional layer in [6], and only a single skip-connection from the input to output is created in the VDSR network. This connection learns the difference between the input and output and prevents the vanishing gradient problem. To expedite the training convergence, a high learning rate is used together with an adjustable gradient clipping scheme where the gradients are clipped to $\left[-\frac{\theta}{\gamma}, \frac{\theta}{\gamma}\right]$ to boost the convergence, where γ denotes the current learning rate and θ is the parameter for gradient clipping.

The structure of the MAC network follows the VDSR network, which comprises 20 convolutional layers and 19 ReLU nonlinear activation functions (Fig. 4). We used 64 filters of the size 3×3 for each convolutional layer. For the corresponding cross-phase style-transferred patch $\tilde{\mathbf{P}}_j^\phi$ is assigned as the GT output for the input patch $\mathbf{P}_j^\phi$, the loss function is defined as the mean squared error $\frac{1}{2}||(\tilde{\mathbf{P}}_j^\phi - \mathbf{P}_j^\phi) - f(\mathbf{P}_j^\phi)||^2$, where f denotes the network prediction of the residual between $\tilde{\mathbf{P}}_j^\phi$ and $\mathbf{P}_j^\phi$. Subsequently, the final result of the network becomes $f(\mathbf{P}_j^\phi) + \mathbf{P}_j^\phi$.

We used the Caffe [10] framework for our implementation. The hyperparameters for training are set as follows: batch size of 64, learning rate of 0.0001, and weight decay of 0.0001. The optimizer 'Adam' [12] is used.

The MAC network can be applied as follows. We assumed that a 3D CT volume of the coronary artery corrupted by motion artifacts is provided. From this volume, we extract the centerline of the coronary artery, sample M equidistant 3D point coordinates, and construct M patches, each centered at these points with normal direction as the centerline tangent direction, similarly as described in Sect. 2.1. All patches are fed into the trained MAC network, separately, where the output patches should have reduced motion artifacts.

3   Experimental Results

3.1   Datasets

In our experiments, we sampled a different number of phases from 100 4D CT volumes because some 3D volumes were excluded where the coronary artery could not be manually identified owing to extremely severe motion artifacts. A total of 5,868 mid-RCA patches were constructed. After a data augmentation process, including vertical and horizontal flips and rotation, the final training set contained a total of 35, 208 patch pairs. Each patch was constructed to be of size 60×60 when sampled from the 3D volume.

For validation, 2547 mid-RCA patches were extracted from 40 4D CT volumes and a total of 15,282 patches were constructed after a data augmentation. For testing, a total of 100 patches, extracted from 10 4D CT volumes, were used.

3.2   Qualitative Evaluation

The outputs of the trained MAC Net are presented in Fig. 5. After applying the proposed method, the edge of the coronary artery is visibly sharper than before. In addition, Fig. 6 shows that the proposed method can compensate the motion artifacts when the coronary artery diverges or contains plaques.

Two experienced readers evaluated the degree of motion artifacts based on a 5-point Likert scale as follows [2]: 1 = completely unreadable; 2 = significant motion; 3 = apparent motion; 4 = minor motion; 5 = no motion. The categorical variables are presented as the ratio of frequencies (see Table 1). The proportion of images presented with completely unreadable, significant, and apparent motions (Likert scale 1, 2, and 3) were 98.5% previously, and decreased to 35% for the MAC Net.

The mean score of the motion artifact is described as mean ± standard deviation. It was significantly improved from 1.43 (± 0.66) to 3.80 (± 0.87). ($p < 0.001$). The inter-observer agreement was calculated with the kappa (κ) statistics for the motion score and it shows a strong agreement: Before ($\kappa = 0.85$; 95% CI 0.76–0.95) and After ($\kappa = 0.70$; 95% CI 0.61–0.81).

4   Discussion

We proposed a motion compensation method of coronary artery in CT images based on deep learning. The key idea of the proposed method is to generate the synthetic motion compensated ground-truth by adopting the neural style-transfer method [5] using full-phase 4D CT images. It enables the patch with motion artifacts to mimic the style of the patches with small artifacts while

Table 1. Motion artifact before and after applying proposed method

	Before	After	p-value
Likert scale			<0.001
1 = Completely unreadable	66.5%	2.5%	
2 = Significant motion	26%	2.5%	
3 = Apparent motion	6%	30%	
4 = Minor motion	1.5%	41.5%	
5 = No motion	0%	23.5%	
Score			<0.001
Mean	1.43	3.80	
Standard deviation	±0.66	±0.87	
Interobserver agreement			
Kappa value	0.85	0.70	
Standard error	±0.05	±0.05	
95% CI	0.76–0.95	0.61–0.81	

retaining its content. The results of the proposed method improved qualitative readability scores from 1.43 to 3.80 on a 5-point Likert score.

While the proposed method showed improved results, in terms of the Likert score, for most cases, there were rare cases where there was no change in the score, as shown in Fig. 7. We assume that motion artifacts are too severe, or the coronary artery is too close to the right atrium or the right ventricle to distinguish its boundary from them. We note that there were no cases where the score decreased, so while there is a possibility that the proposed method does no good, there is very little possibility that it will do harm.

For future work, we intend to address the re-projection of the output patches into the original 3D CT volume and volumetric interpolation. This process is required to analyze the coronary artery in commercial software in practice. Further, we expect to quantify the motion artifacts based on the metric system and compare the performances before and after applying the proposed method. We also hope to use the quantitative measurements to perform comparative analysis with previous methods based on retrospective motion compensation based on motion estimation.

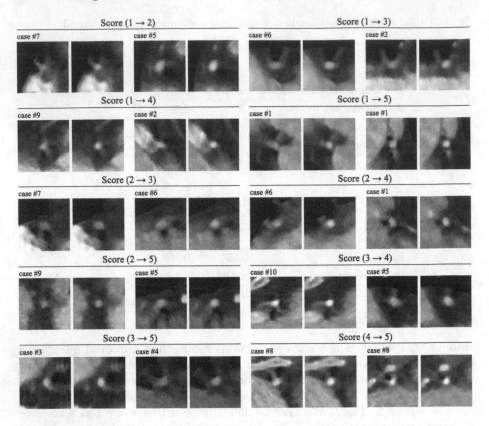

Fig. 5. Qualitative results of the test datasets. Left and right in each dataset mean before and after applying the proposed method, respectively. Expert evaluated scores based on 5-point Likert scale [2] and case number are presented above each dataset.

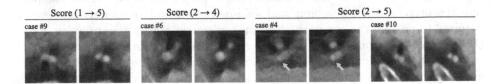

Fig. 6. Qualitative results of specific cases that distinguish well the primary vessel from the branch. The third sample pair also shows compensation for the artery plaque. Left and right in each dataset mean before and after applying the proposed method, respectively. Expert evaluated scores and case number are presented above.

Score (1 → 1) Score (2 → 2)

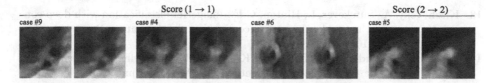

Fig. 7. Qualitative results of specific cases with little changes in motion artifacts. Left and right in each dataset mean before and after applying the proposed method, respectively. Expert evaluated scores and case number are presented above.

Acknowledgment. This research was supported by the National Research Foundation of Korea (NRF) funded by the Ministry of Science, ICT & Future Planning (MSIP) (2012027176) and (NRF-2015R1C1A1A01054697).

References

1. Bhagalia, R., Pack, J.D., Miller, J.V., Iatrou, M.: Nonrigid registration-based coronary artery motion correction for cardiac computed tomography. Med. Phys. **39**(7), 4245–4254 (2012)
2. Cho, I., et al.: Heart-rate dependent improvement in image quality and diagnostic accuracy of coronary computed tomographic angiography by novel intracycle motion correction algorithm. Clin. Imaging **39**(3), 421–426 (2015)
3. Collobert, R., Weston, J.: A unified architecture for natural language processing: deep neural networks with multitask learning. In: Proceedings of the 25th International Conference on Machine Learning, pp. 160–167. ACM (2008)
4. Deng, J., Dong, W., Socher, R., Li, L.J., Li, K., Fei-Fei, L.: ImageNet: a large-scale hierarchical image database. In: 2009 IEEE Conference on Computer Vision and Pattern Recognition, CVPR 2009, pp. 248–255. IEEE (2009)
5. Gatys, L.A., Ecker, A.S., Bethge, M.: A neural algorithm of artistic style. arXiv preprint arXiv:1508.06576 (2015)
6. He, K., Zhang, X., Ren, S., Sun, J.: Deep residual learning for image recognition. In: Proceedings of the IEEE Conference on Computer Vision and Pattern Recognition, pp. 770–778 (2016)
7. Heron, M.P.: Deaths: leading causes for 2012. National Vital Statistics Reports (2015)
8. Hinton, G.: Deep neural networks for acoustic modeling in speech recognition: the shared views of four research groups. IEEE Sig. Process. Mag. **29**(6), 82–97 (2012)
9. Isola, A.A., Grass, M., Niessen, W.J.: Fully automatic nonrigid registration-based local motion estimation for motion-corrected iterative cardiac CT reconstruction. Med. Phys. **37**(3), 1093–1109 (2010)
10. Jia, Y., et al.: Caffe: convolutional architecture for fast feature embedding. In: Proceedings of the 22nd ACM International Conference on Multimedia, pp. 675–678. ACM (2014)
11. Kim, J., Lee, J.K., Lee, K.M.: Accurate image super-resolution using very deep convolutional networks. In: Proceedings of the IEEE Conference on Computer Vision and Pattern Recognition, pp. 1646–1654 (2016)
12. Kingma, D., Ba, J.: Adam: a method for stochastic optimization. arXiv preprint arXiv:1412.6980 (2014)

13. Krizhevsky, A., Sutskever, I., Hinton, G.E.: ImageNet classification with deep convolutional neural networks. In: Advances in Neural Information Processing Systems, pp. 1097–1105 (2012)
14. Rohkohl, C., Bruder, H., Stierstorfer, K., Flohr, T.: Improving best-phase image quality in cardiac CT by motion correction with MAM optimization. Med. Phys. **40**(3), 031901 (2013)
15. Simonyan, K., Zisserman, A.: Very deep convolutional networks for large-scale image recognition. arXiv preprint arXiv:1409.1556 (2014)
16. Tang, Q., Cammin, J., Srivastava, S., Taguchi, K.: A fully four-dimensional, iterative motion estimation and compensation method for cardiac CT. Med. Phys. **39**(7), 4291–4305 (2012)
17. Vincent, P., Larochelle, H., Lajoie, I., Bengio, Y., Manzagol, P.A.: Stacked denoising autoencoders: learning useful representations in a deep network with a local denoising criterion. J. Mach. Learn. Res. **11**(Dec), 3371–3408 (2010)

Lung Nodule Synthesis Using CNN-Based Latent Data Representation

Dario Augusto Borges Oliveira[✉] and Matheus Palhares Viana

IBM Research Brazil, Rua Tutóia, 1157, Paraíso, São Paulo, Brazil
darioaugusto@gmail.com

Abstract. Convolutional neural networks (CNNs) have been widely used to address various image analysis problems at the cost of intensive computational load and large amounts of annotated training data. When it comes to Medical Imaging, annotation is often complicated and/or expensive, and innovative methods for dealing with small or very imbalanced training sets are mostly welcome. In this context, this paper proposes a novel approach for efficiently synthesizing volumetric patch data from a small amount of samples using their latent data. Our method consists of two major steps. First, we train a 3D CNN autoencoder for unsupervised learning of volumetric latent data by means of multivariate Gaussian mixture models (GMMs): while the encoder finds latent representations of volumes using GMMs, the decoder uses the estimated GMMs parameters to reconstruct the volume observed in the input. Then, we modify latent data of samples at training time to generate similar, but different, new samples: we run non-rigid registrations between patches decoded from real latent data and patches decoded from modified latent data, and warp the corresponding original image patches using the resulting displacement fields. We evaluated our method in the context of lung nodules synthesis using the publicly available LUNA challenge dataset, and generated new realistic samples out of real lung nodules, preserving their original texture and neighbouring anatomical structures. Our results demonstrate that 3D CNNs trained using our synthesis method were able to consistently deliver lower lung nodule false positive rates, which indicates an improvement in the networks discriminant power.

Keywords: Nodules synthesis · Generative models
Convolutional neural networks
Multivariate Gaussian mixture models
Lung nodule false positive reduction

1 Introduction

Convolutional neural networks (CNNs) have been successfully used for image analysis in a number of different applications. In medical imaging they support image segmentation and classification, exams retrieval, and aid in diagnosis,

© Springer Nature Switzerland AG 2018
A. Gooya et al. (Eds.): SASHIMI 2018, LNCS 11037, pp. 111–118, 2018.
https://doi.org/10.1007/978-3-030-00536-8_12

helping specialists to analyze more exams in less time with higher precision. Extensive reviews of deep learning applied to medical imaging are available in the literature [3,6].

CNNs usually rely on heavy computation and huge loads of training data to deliver outstanding results. Since creating training data in medicine is usually non-trivial and/or very expensive, an ongoing discussion in the medical imaging community concerns empowering these networks with capabilities that allow their use in small training datasets. In this scenario, innovative data augmentation methods have received growing attention in the community in the last few years.

This paper presents a novel data augmentation method that creates rich volumetric patch data from a small amount of samples using their latent data representation. We propose a two major steps approach: first, we use an auto-encoder architecture to perform unsupervised learning of a mixture of multivariate Gaussian distributions to model lung nodules; then, we apply perturbations to latent data to generate similar but different new samples, through a simple non-rigid registration that roughly preserves their texture and neighbouring anatomical structures. With this simple but powerful pipeline we deliver rich data augmentation in training time.

To evaluate our approach, we used the publicly available LUNA challenge dataset and demonstrate that the proposed data synthesis method allows CNNs to improve lung nodule classification accuracy, with a clear benefit from using the synthetically created data for training. Our report includes results from 3D CNNs trained with usual data augmentation techniques and results from a very common benchmark for lung nodule false positive reduction. Comparison to many other methods is straightforward in the extensive compile of LUNA challenge [5].

The remainder of this paper is organized as follows: in Sect. 2 we describe the proposed pipeline consisting of our latent data extraction method and the non-rigid registration schema used for generating realistic synthetic samples. Then, we describe our experiments in Sect. 3 and present our results and discussions in Sect. 4. Finally, conclusions are drawn in Sect. 5.

2   Methodology

Tools for aid in lung nodules diagnosis commonly use image processing techniques to generate a large number of candidates for nodules location [5]. A candidate is represented by its position in 3D and is given a label, for instance $\ell_q \in [0,1]$, that identifies a false or true nodule. Classification methods are used to filter the list of candidates and narrow it down to strong candidates that should be visually inspected by a specialist. An usual bottleneck happens when the number of false nodule candidates to be checked (false positives) is too high. In this context, LUNA challenge proposed a track to foster the development of methods for lung nodule false positive reduction.

The challenge compile presented in [5] highlighted that many methods struggled with the imbalanced nature of this problem: in a dataset of nearly 750.000

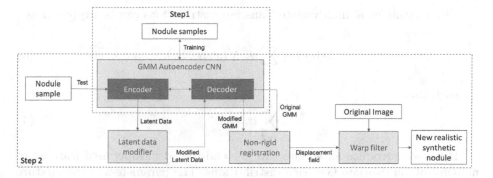

Fig. 1. Our two-step approach: first we extract the nodules latent data representation using a GMM auto-encoder CNN; then we use the CNN output to generate new realistic nodules using a non-rigid registration schema.

candidates, only around 2.000 are true nodules. 3D convolution networks deliver the state-of-art in the false positive reduction track, and data augmentation methods were widely used to cope with this severe data imbalance.

In this paper we perform data augmentation using a synthesis method that creates new realistic samples out of the available nodules training set. As shown in Fig. 1, our method is composed by two steps: first, we extract the nodules latent data representation; then, we use them to generate new realistic nodules using a non-rigid registration schema. Each of these steps is explained in the following.

2.1   GMM Latent Data Representation

Mixture models are conveniently used to describe systems composed by sub-populations within an overall population. Gaussian mixture models (GMM) in particular, are widely applied to different areas, ranging from speaker recognition to image retrieval, finance, electron and atomic position, spectroscopy, cellular components. GMM has also been shown to be useful for modeling colour features in order to classify coloured textures in images [4]. Herein, we propose to model lung nodules as GMM models to extract their latent data representation.

The n-dimensional multivariate Gaussian distributions is written as

$$\mathcal{N}(\boldsymbol{x}, \boldsymbol{\mu}, \boldsymbol{\Sigma}) = \frac{1}{\sqrt{2\pi\boldsymbol{\Sigma}}} \exp\left[-\frac{1}{2}(\boldsymbol{x}-\boldsymbol{\mu})^T \boldsymbol{\Sigma}^{-1}(\boldsymbol{x}-\boldsymbol{\mu})\right], \tag{1}$$

where $\boldsymbol{\mu}$ is the mean and $\boldsymbol{\Sigma}$ is the positive-definite covariance matrix

$$\boldsymbol{\Sigma} = \begin{bmatrix} \sigma_1^2 & \rho_{1,2}\sigma_1\sigma_2 \cdots \\ \vdots & \ddots \\ \rho_{n,1}\sigma_n\sigma_1 & \sigma_n^2 \end{bmatrix}. \tag{2}$$

The mixture of K multivariate Gaussian distributions can be expressed as

$$\mathcal{M}(\boldsymbol{x}) = \sum_{i=1}^{K} \alpha_i \, \mathcal{N}(\boldsymbol{x}, \boldsymbol{\mu}_i, \boldsymbol{\Sigma}_i), \tag{3}$$

such that

$$\sum_{i=1}^{K} \alpha_i = 1. \tag{4}$$

Here, we introduce an architecture for end-to-end unsupervised learning of mixture of multivariate Gaussian distributions. The parameters of the mixture are learned from a latent representation of the input data and used to reconstruct the input using Eq. 1. A convolutional encoder is used to create a latent representation $\boldsymbol{y}$ for n−dimensional input data $\boldsymbol{x}$, with $n = 3$, according to

$$\boldsymbol{y} = \Phi\left(\mathbf{W}_0 \boldsymbol{x} + \boldsymbol{b}_0\right). \tag{5}$$

The latent representation $\boldsymbol{y}$, which is of size $\ell \times 1$, is then used as input for dense layers that estimate the parameters α_i, $\boldsymbol{\mu}_i$ and $\boldsymbol{\Sigma}_i$, $0 \leq i \leq K$. Because of the constraint expressed in Eq. 4, we use softmax activation for estimating $\alpha's$. We used tanh for estimating the mean vector of each component, which lie in the range $[-1, 1]$ representing the domain of the input data. Standard deviation and correlation parameters are estimated through sigmoid activation and they are composed to build the covariance matrices given by Eq. 2. Therefore, the parameters of our mixture model can be expressed as

$$\boldsymbol{\alpha} = softmax\left(\mathbf{W}_1 \boldsymbol{y} + \boldsymbol{b}_1\right), \tag{6}$$

$$\boldsymbol{\mu}_1, \ldots, \boldsymbol{\mu}_K = tanh\left(\mathbf{W}_2 \boldsymbol{y} + \boldsymbol{b}_2\right), \tag{7}$$

$$\boldsymbol{\sigma}_1, \ldots, \boldsymbol{\sigma}_K = sigmoid\left(\mathbf{W}_3 \boldsymbol{y} + \boldsymbol{b}_3\right), \tag{8}$$

$$\rho_{1,2}^{(1)}, \ldots, \rho_{n-1,n}^{(K)} = sigmoid\left(\mathbf{W}_4 \boldsymbol{y} + \boldsymbol{b}_4\right). \tag{9}$$

In total, our architecture estimates $1/2(n^2 + 3n + 2)K$ parameters from the latent representation of the input data. The last layer in our architecture uses the estimated parameters to create the n-dimensional density map in Eq. 3. The resulting density map is compared to the input data according to a loss function of our choice (we used the logarithm of the hyperbolic cosine of the prediction error), and visual results of the training process are shown in Fig. 2-I. In our experiments, we used 16×16x16 patches and experimentally defined $K = 50$.

2.2   Sample Synthesis Using Non-rigid Registration

For new samples synthesis, we used the trained encoder to compute the latent data representation of a given real nodule, and used it as a model for creating new samples, as shown in Fig. 1.

Since we trained our decoder to map latent data representation into GMMs, we could create reasonable new GMMs by simply adding noise to the latent

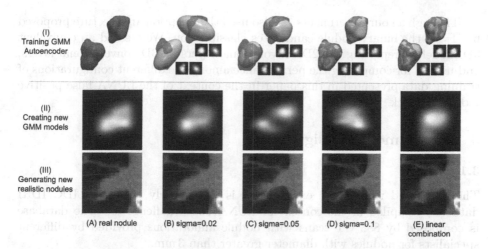

Fig. 2. In (I) we show the visual outcome of step 1: training the GMM autoencoder. In (II) and (III) we show the visual outcome of step 2: creating GMM models in (II), and generating realistic nodules in (III). From (A) to (E) we show different configurations of the proposed methodology.

data or an applying a linear combination of two different latent data vectors, as shown in Fig. 2-II. This way we create new density maps that represent slightly different nodule samples.

Then we used a non-rigid deformation approach for creating realistic samples that respect boundaries transitions and surrounding anatomical structures. We take the density volume reconstructed using the original latent data and use it as the moving image of a Level Sets motion registration filter (implementation provided by SimpleITK [7]) targeting the density volume generated by the modified latent data as fixed image. Finally, we warp the original image using the resulting displacement field, and deform the original sample creating a new and realistic sample.

This simple schema allow us to create diverse synthetic samples, and control at some extension, the heterogeneity rate observed in the process, as shown in Fig. 2-III. For completeness, we used 50 iterations and a gradient smoothing standard deviations in the Level Set filters, all other parameters set as default in SimpleITK.

2.3   CNN Architectures

The GMM auto-encoder architecture herein proposed consisted of an encoder composed of 3 convolutional layers with $32 \times 7 \times 7, 32 \times 5 \times 5$ and $32 \times 3 \times 3$ filters respectively, and a dense layer with 516 nodes, which holds sample latent data representation; and a decoder that receives the latent data and decodes it into dense layers α_i, μ_i and Σ_i, $0 \leq i \leq K$ used to reconstruct the volume targeting the input sample.

Through all our experiments we also used the Xception architecture proposed by [1] for the binary nodule candidates classification. We created an equivalent 3D model by replacing the 2D convolutional layers by 3D convolutional layers, and used it for comparing the performance among the different configurations of training data presented in this paper in the context of the LUNA false positive reduction track.

3   Experiments Design

3.1   Data

The data used through all experiments is the publicly available LIDC/IDRI database compiled in the context of LUNA 2016 challenge [5]. The database is composed by 888 CT scans with nodule annotations provided by different specialists for nodules with diameter greater than 3 mm.

As pre-processing for nodule candidates classification, we extracted 3D patches from the CT exams in three different scales: 10 mm × 10 mm × 10 mm, 25 mm × 25 mm × 25 mm and 40 mm × 40 mm × 40 mm, each of them sampled as 50 × 50 × 50 patches. Each scale was represented as a different channel, meaning that final 3D patches have 50 × 50 × 50 × 3 voxels. For nodule data augmentation using our synthesis method, the deformation field was applied to the corresponding region in each scale.

3.2   Training and Testing Procedures

For training the GMM auto-encoder, we selected all the available nodules (around 2100 samples) and resized them to 16 × 16 × 16 patches. We trained the model until the loss error was 5×10^{-5} or less, which was achieved after around 500 epochs. Then, we used the trained network to generate latent data to be further modified to generate new realistic nodules.

The CNN models for false positive reduction were trained using the cross-validation schema proposed in LUNA challenge. The organization provided an available dataset divided into 10 different subsets, and for each fold we used nine subsets for training, and the remaining one for testing the trained model. In our experiments, we used 1 subset of the training data for validation and Adam for weights optimization. We trained all classification models using two sequences of 20 epochs, and augmented the nodule class samples using either synthetic nodules created by our method or random rotations, and sub-sampled at random the non-nodule class to balance the training dataset, comprising a total of 75000 samples per epoch evenly balanced. During the test we did not use any synthetic data.

4   Results and Discussion

Our experiments highlight the benefits of using the proposed synthetic data augmentation for lung nodules false positive reduction. We executed five different experiments: one benchmark using simple rotations as data augmentation for training data, three experiments adding noise to the latent data representation using normal distributions with different standard deviations ($sigma = [0.02, 0.05, 0.1]$), and a last experiment that modifies the latent data using a linear combination ($0.5 * (y_1 + y_2)$) of two different latent data arrays. We evaluated the accuracy in terms of false positive reduction ROC curves. Note that the analysis of other CNN architectures and the extensive analysis of parameters in the Xception architecture could potentially improve results, but this was beyond our objectives in this paper.

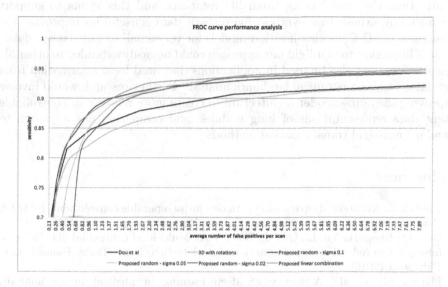

Fig. 3. FROC curves representing the performance of different configurations of our proposed data augmentation method, an usual 3D data augmentation method and the available state-of-art in the literature.

Our results demonstrate that our method delivers considerable superior performance for all tested configurations when compared with usual rotations for 3D patches augmentation and a very common benchmark [2] in the literature, as shown in Fig. 3. Note that other methods with better performance are available in the challenge website but most of them do not have a peer reviewed paper associated, so we do not compare to them. We observed an **increase of 5.86%@2FP** in sensitivity when compared to regular data augmentation training. It is also interesting to notice that increasing *sigma* improves the performance of the corresponding CNN, meaning that more heterogeneous data increases the classification network robustness, as expected. It is also remarkable that the linear combination of two latent data representations achieved the best overall performance in the tested models. This reinforces the idea that increasing the heterogeneity of training nodules leads to more robust CNN models, but at the same time highlights that combining latent data of real nodules probably derive more realistic samples, as observed in Fig. 2-D/E.

5   Conclusions

This paper presents an innovative method for synthesizing new realistic samples out of real lung nodules. We evaluated our method using the LUNA challenge false positive reduction track, and our results point to a clear benefit of augmenting training data using our approach. All tested configurations delivered better results than the model using usual 3D rotations, and this seems to support our initial hypothesis that synthesizing realistic data is useful for improving the robustness of 3D CNN classification models for very small or imbalanced data.

It is important to highlight our approach could be easily extended to other 3D image exams, and also be used in applications that need local information from few data, such as anatomical landmark analysis. Further research would involve improving the auto-encoder architecture to create more realistic or controllable latent data representations of lung nodules, and comparing our approach to standard non-rigid transformation methods.

References

1. Chollet, F.: Xception: deep learning with depthwise separable convolutions. In: IEEE Conference on Computer Vision and Pattern Recognition, pp. 1251–1258 (2017)
2. Dou, Q., Chen, H., Yu, L., Qin, J., Heng, P.A.: Multi-level contextual 3D CNNs for false positive reduction in pulmonary nodule detection. IEEE Trans. Biomed. Eng. **PP**(99), 1 (2016)
3. Litjens, G., et al.: A survey on deep learning in medical image analysis. Med. Image Anal. **42**(Suppl. C), 60–88 (2017). http://www.sciencedirect.com/science/article/pii/S1361841517301135
4. Permuter, H., Francos, J., Jermyn, I.H.: Gaussian mixture models of texture and colour for image database retrieval. In: 2003 IEEE International Conference on Acoustics, Speech, and Signal Processing, Proceedings (ICASSP 2003), vol. 3, p. III-569. IEEE (2003)
5. Setio, A.A.A.: Validation, comparison, and combination of algorithms for automatic detection of pulmonary nodules in computed tomography images: the LUNA16 challenge. Med. Image Anal. **42**, 1–13 (2017). https://doi.org/10.1016/j.media.2017.06.015
6. Tajbakhsh, N., et al.: Convolutional neural networks for medical image analysis: full training or fine tuning? IEEE Trans. Med. Imaging **35**(5), 1299–1312 (2016)
7. Yaniv, Z., Lowekamp, B.C., Johnson, H.J., Beare, R.: SimpleITK image-analysis notebooks: a collaborative environment for education and reproducible research. J. Digit. Imaging (2017). https://doi.org/10.1007/s10278-017-0037-8

RS-Net: Regression-Segmentation 3D CNN for Synthesis of Full Resolution Missing Brain MRI in the Presence of Tumours

Raghav Mehta[✉] and Tal Arbel

McGill University, Montreal, QC, Canada
raghav@cim.mcgill.ca

Abstract. Accurate synthesis of a full 3D MR image containing tumours from available MRI (e.g. to replace an image that is currently unavailable or corrupted) would provide a clinician as well as downstream inference methods with important complementary information for disease analysis. In this paper, we present an end-to-end 3D convolution neural network that takes a set of acquired MR image sequences (e.g. T1, T2, T1ce) as input and concurrently performs (1) regression of the missing full resolution 3D MRI (e.g. FLAIR) and (2) segmentation of the tumour into subtypes (e.g. enhancement, core). The hypothesis is that this would focus the network to perform accurate synthesis in the area of the tumour. Experiments on the BraTS 2015 and 2017 datasets [1] show that: (1) the proposed method gives better performance than state-of-the art methods in terms of established global evaluation metrics (e.g. PSNR), (2) replacing real MR volumes with the synthesized MRI does not lead to significant degradation in tumour and sub-structure segmentation accuracy. The system further provides uncertainty estimates based on Monte Carlo (MC) dropout [11] for the synthesized volume at each voxel, permitting quantification of the system's confidence in the output at each location.

Keywords: Deep learning · Image synthesis · Brain MRI

1 Introduction

The presence of a variety of different Magnetic Resonance (MR) sequences (e.g. T1, T2, Fluid Attenuated Inverse Recovery (FLAIR)) improves the analysis in the context of neurological diseases such as multiple sclerosis and brain cancers, because different sequences provide complementary information. In particular, the accuracy of detection and segmentation of lesions and tumours greatly increases should several sequences of MR be available [2], as different sequences assist in differentiating healthy tissues from focal pathologies. However, in real clinical practice, not all MR image sequences are always available for each patient

© Springer Nature Switzerland AG 2018
A. Gooya et al. (Eds.): SASHIMI 2018, LNCS 11037, pp. 119–129, 2018.
https://doi.org/10.1007/978-3-030-00536-8_13

for a variety of reasons, including cost or time constraints, or at times, images are available but not usable, for example due to corruption from noise or patient motion. As such, both clinical practice and automatic segmentation techniques would benefit greatly from the synthesis of one or more of the missing 3D MR image sequences based on the others provided [3]. However, synthesis of full 3D brain MR image is challenging especially in the presence of pathology as different MR sequences represent pathology in a different way.

Recently, modality synthesis has gained some attention from the medical image analysis community [4–6]. Several approaches have been explored, such as patch-based random forest [4] and sparse dictionary reconstruction [5]. Regression Ensembles with Patch Learning for Image Contrast Agreement (REPLICA) [4] was developed to synthesize T2-weighted MRI from T1-weighted MRI using the bagged ensemble of random forests based on nonlinear patch regression. Given the success of Convolutional Neural Networks (CNNs) [7] and Generative Adversarial Networks (GANs) [8] for image-to-image translation in the field of computer vision, several recent 2D CNN [6,9] and 2D GANs [10] have been developed for modality synthesis in the context of medical imaging, showing promising results for synthesis of healthy subject MRI. A patch-based Location Sensitive Deep Network (LSDN) [6] was developed to combine intensity and spatial information for synthesizing T2 MRI from T1 MRI and vice versa. A 2D CNN model was developed to generate 2D synthesized images with missing input MRI [9]. Quantitative analysis showed superior performance over competing methods based on global image metrics (PSNR and SSIM). However, the performance of the method in the area of focal pathology was not examined.

In this paper, an end-to-end 3D CNN is developed that takes as input a set of acquired MRI sequences of patients with tumours and simultaneously performs (1) regression to generate a full resolution missing 3D MR modality and (2) segmentation of the brain tumour into subtypes. The hypothesis is that by performing regression and segmentation concurrently, the network should produce full-resolution, high quality 3D MR images, particularly the area of the tumour. The network is trained and tested on the MICCAI 2015 and 2017 BraTS datasets [1]. In the first set of experiments, the framework is evaluated against state-of-the-art synthesis methods [4,6,9] based on global image metrics used in previous work [9], where it is shown to slightly outperform all reported results. The second set of experiments evaluate the synthesis quality at pathological locations, by examining its performance on subsequent independent downstream tasks, namely tumour segmentation. Results show that real MR images can be swapped with the generated synthesized T1, T2, and FLAIR MR images with minimal loss in segmentation performance. The network also quantifies the uncertainty of the regressed synthetic volumes through Monte Carlo dropout [11]. This permits the confidence in the synthesis results to be conveyed to radiologists and clinicians and to automatic downstream methods that would use the synthesized volumes as inputs.

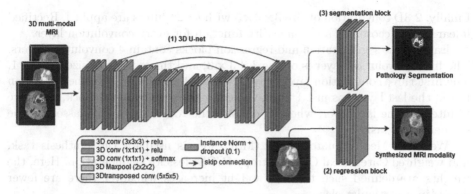

Fig. 1. Proposed Regression-Segmentation CNN architecture (RS-Net): (1) A 3D U-net, (2) Regression and (3) Segmentation convolution blocks. The model takes as input several full 3D MR image sequences, synthesizes the missing 3D MRI, while concurrently generating the multi-class segmentation of the tumour into sub-types.

2 Regression-Segmentation CNN Architecture

A flowchart of the proposed Regression-Segmentation CNN architecture (**RS-Net**) can be seen in Fig. 1. The network consists of three main components: (1) a modified 3D U-net [12], (2) regression convolution block for synthesizing image sequence, and (3) segmentation convolution block for multi-class tumour segmentation. RS-Net takes as input full 3D volumes of all available sequences of a patient. The U-net generates an intermediate latent representation of the inputs which is provided to the regression and the segmentation convolution blocks. These then generate synthesis of the missing 3D MR image sequences and multi-class segmentation of tumours into sub-types, at the same resolution. The U-net learns latent representation which is common to both tumour segmentation and synthesis, with focus on high accuracy in the area containing tumour structures. In addition to the U-net output, the regression block is also provided with one of the input MRIs, which will provide necessary brain MR context to the regression block. The architecture details are now described.

The 3D U-net is similar to the one proposed in [12], with some modifications. The U-net consists of 4 resolution steps for both encoder and decoder paths. At the start, we use 2 consecutive 3D convolutions of size $3 \times 3 \times 3$ with k filters, where k denotes the user-defined initial number of convolution filters. Each step in the encoder path consists of 2 3D convolutions of size $3 \times 3 \times 3$ with $k*2^n$ filters, where n denotes the U-net resolution step. This is followed by maxpooling of size $2 \times 2 \times 2$. At the end of each encoder step, instance normalization [13] is applied, followed by dropout [14] with 0.1 probability. In the decoder path at each step, 3D transposed convolution of size $5 \times 5 \times 5$ is applied, with $2 \times 2 \times 2$ stride and $k*2^n$ filters for the upsampling task. The output of the transposed convolution is concatenated with the corresponding output of the encoder path. This is, once again, followed by instance normalization and Dropout with 0.1 probability.

Finally, 2 3D convolution of size $3 \times 3 \times 3$ with $k * 2^n$ filters are applied. Rectified linear unit is chosen as a non-linearity function for every convolution layer.

Each of the segmentation and regression blocks contain 4 convolution layers. The first convolution layer is of size $3 \times 3 \times 3$, and the rest are of size $1 \times 1 \times 1$. The first three convolution layers have $k * 4$, $k * 2$ and k filters. In the regression block, the last layer has just 1 filter, while, for the segmentation block, there are C filters in the last layer, where C denotes the total number of classes for the segmentation task.

Weighted Mean Squared Error (MSE) loss is used for the synthesis task, and weighted Categorical Cross Entropy (CCE) loss for segmentation. Here, the weights are defined such that the weight increases whenever there are fewer voxels in a particular class.

$$w_n^i = w_l * y_n^i \qquad \text{where, } w_l = \left(\frac{\sum_{k=0}^{k=C} m_k}{m_l} \right) * r^{ep} + 1, \qquad (1)$$

where, w_n^i and w_l denote the weight for voxel n of volume i and the weight of class l. m_l is total number of voxels of lth class in the training dataset. w_l are decayed over each epoch ep with a rate of $r \in [0, 1]$. It should be noted that w_l converges to 1 as ep becomes large. The final loss function for the network, L^i, (for volume i) is a weighted combination of both of these loss functions:

$$L^i = \lambda_1(MSE^i) + \lambda_2(CCE^i). \qquad (2)$$

Given the challenges associated with regressing a synthesized volume, errors are bound to exist. As such, deterministic outputs present dangers to subsequent clinical decisions as well as to downstream automatic methods that make use of the results. In this work, the network output is augmented with uncertainty estimates based on Monte Carlo dropout [11]. During testing, N Monte Carlo (MC) samples of the output are acquired by passing each set of input volumes N times through the network to predict N different synthesized output MR volumes with probability of randomly dropping any neuron of the network equal to the dropout rate. Uncertainty in the synthesized volume, during testing, is estimated based on the variance of the MC samples at every voxel.

3   Experiments and Results

We now evaluate the performance of the RS-Net using two sets of experiments. In the first set of experiments, we compare the quality of the synthesized volume generated by RS-Net against other methods [4,6,9] using PSNR and SSIM on 2015 MICCAI BraTS dataset [1]. In the second set of experiments, we evaluate the quality of the synthesized volumes in a downstream task of tumor segmentation on 2017 MICCAI BraTS datasets [1].

RS-Net uses 4 initial convolutional filters and 4 steps for U-net encoder and decoder paths. This results in a network with a total of 674455 learnable parameters. Values of λ_1 and λ_2 in the loss function (Eq. 2), to combine CCE and MSE,

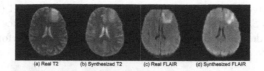

(a) Real T2   (b) Synthesized T2   (c) Real FLAIR   (d) Synthesized FLAIR

Fig. 2. Example slice from synthetic MR volumes generated by the proposed RS-Net on BraTS 2015 dataset for T1-to-T2 and T1-to-FLAIR synthesis.

were fixed to 1.0 and 0.1 respectively based on experimentation evidence. The networks were trained on a NVIDIA Titan Xp GPU for 240 epochs. Approximate training time was 3 days. The networks were trained with batch size of 1, using Adam optimizer [15] with the following hyperparameters: learning rate $= 0.0002$, $\beta_1 = 0.9$, $\beta_2 = 0.999$ and $\epsilon = 10^{-08}$. During testing time, a total of 20 samples of the output were generated to estimate the uncertainty in the synthesized volumes.

3.1 Comparison of RS-Net Synthesis Results Against Other Methods

In order to compare the quality of the synthesized volumes produced by RS-Net against other state-of-the-art methods, namely REPLICA [4], LSDN [6], and 2D CNN [9], we train two different RS-Nets for T2 and FLAIR synthesis from T1 MRI, as done by Chartsias et al. [9]. We use the evaluation metrics, SSIM [16] and PSNR, defined in [9], to evaluate the quality of the synthesized volumes.

Given a ground-truth volume X and its corresponding synthesized volume $\hat{X}$, SSIM is computed as $SSIM(X, \hat{X}) = \frac{(2\mu_X \mu_{\hat{X}} + c_1)(2\sigma_{X\hat{X}} + c_2)}{(\mu_X^2 + \mu_{\hat{X}}^2 + c_1)(\sigma_X^2 + \sigma_{\hat{X}}^2 + c_1)}$, where μ_X and σ_X^2 are mean and variance of volume X and $\sigma_{X\hat{X}}$ is the covariance between X and $\hat{X}$. PSNR is computed as $10 \log_{10}(\frac{MAX_I^2}{MSE})$ where MAX_I is the maximum intensity of the volume and MSE is the mean squared error between volumes X and $\hat{X}$.

In order to compare our results to those in the paper [9], experiments were performed on the 2015 MICCAI BraTS training dataset [1]. This dataset consists of High-Grade Glioma (HGG) and Low-Grade Glioma (LGG) cases. 54 LGG cases were acquired with T1, T2, T1ce, and FLAIR. Four tumour subclasses were defined. Volumes are skull-stripped, co-registered, and interpolated to $1 \, mm^3$ voxel dimension. Each volume is of size $240 \times 240 \times 155$. We follow the same pre-processing steps followed in [9], where we normalize each volume by dividing by the volume's average intensity. Following [9], we perform 5-fold cross validation on the dataset (LGG cases). Here, for each cross-validation fold, the dataset is divided into three sets, namely, training, validation, and testing. Each set consists of 42, 6, and 6 volumes respectively.

Quantitative comparison of all different methods is given in Table 1. It should be noted that we didn't reproduce the results for other methods and instead report them as listed in [9]. Results indicate that RS-Net performs slightly better

Table 1. Quantitative results for T1-to-T2 (top) and T1-to-FLAIR (bottom) synthesis based on PSNR and SSIM. Higher values indicate better performance. Values in bracket represent standard deviation across volumes. Absolute highest performing results seen in bold.

	REPLICA [4]	LSDN [6]	2D-CNN [9]	RS-Net (proposed)
T2				
SSMI	0.901 (0.01)	0.909 (0.02)	0.929 (0.17)	**0.934 (0.02)**
PSNR	28.62 (1.69)	30.12 (1.62)	30.96 (1.85)	**31.13 (1.78)**
FLAIR				
SSMI	0.870 (0.01)	0.887 (0.01)	0.897 (0.01)	**0.900 (0.01)**
PSNR	28.32 (1.38)	29.68 (1.56)	30.32 (1.61)	**30.88 (1.84)**

than other methods based on the global metrics of PSNR and SSIM, for both T1-to-T2 and T1-to-FLAIR synthesis. The results also show the advantage of using the proposed 3D CNN over 2D CNN. An example showing qualitative results based on RS-Net for both T2 and FLAIR synthesis on a testing volume is shown in Fig. 2. Note that the resulting MR images are visually similar to the real images, particularly in the area of the tumour.

3.2 Evaluation of RS-Net Synthesis Results on Downstream Tumour Segmentation Task

The metrics used in the previous section can be useful in assessing global synthesis quality, but in the context of volumes with pathological structures such as lesions or tumours synthesis quality assessment should focus on the pathological areas. To this end, we quantitatively evaluate the synthesis performance based on their effect on downstream method, tumour segmentation and tumour sub-class segmentation. To this end, we train a new segmentation CNN, for the specific task of multi-class tumor segmentation (referred to as **S-Net**). This network is similar to the RS-Net but modified such that the synthesis convolution block is removed. S-Net is trained using all 4 real MR volumes with weighted CCE as the loss function. To evaluate the quality of the synthesized volume, one of the real MR volumes is swapped with the synthesized one and the segmentation accuracy is measured. Note that we do <u>not</u> retrain the S-Net with the synthesized volume. This allows us to measure quality of the synthesized volumes in comparison to the real volumes.

Dataset and Pre-processing: The 2017 MICCAI BraTS [1] datasets were used for all the experiments in this section. The BraTS training dataset was used to train the networks. This dataset is comprised of 210 HGG and 75 LGG patients with T1, T1 post contrast (T1ce), T2, and FLAIR MRI for each patient, along with expert tumor labels for each of 3 classes: edema, necrotic/non-enhancing core, and enhancing tumor core. 228 volumes were randomly selected

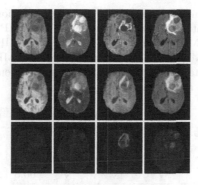

Fig. 3. Example slice from synthetic MR volumes generated using the proposed RS-Net along with its associated uncertainties. Real MRI (Row 1); synthesized volumes (Row 2) and its associated uncertainty (Row 3) produced as mean and variance across 20 MC dropout samples. Columns from left to right: T1, T2, T1ce, and FLAIR. Notice that uncertainties are highest where predicted tumour enhancements in T1ce are incorrect.

for training the network and another remaining 57 for network validation. A separate BraTS 2017 validation dataset, held out during training, was used to test the synthesis and segmentation performance. This dataset contains 46 patient multi-channel MRI (with no labels provided). The BraTS challenge provided pre-processed volumes that were skull-stripped, co-aligned, and resampled to $1\,mm^3$ voxel volume. The intensities were additionally rescaled using mean subtraction, divided by the standard deviation, and rescaled from 0 to 1 and were cropped to $184 \times 200 \times 152$. For this context, the additional complementary input presented to the regression block (see Fig. 1(3)) for T1, T2, T1ce, and FLAIR sequences were T1ce, FLAIR, T1, and T2 respectively. This was chosen as T1ce is the gadolinium enhanced version of T1, and FLAIR is the fluid attenuated version of T2.

Qualitative Evaluation: Synthesis MR volumes produced in a leave-one-out approach by 4 different RS-Nets such that three real MR sequences are used to synthesize the fourth (see Fig. 3). The results indicate that the network is able to produce high-quality, high-resolution, 3D synthesized MR volumes, particularly for T1 and T2 sequences, and even for FLAIR. As T1ce shows enhancement within the tumour based on injection of a contrast agent, it was not expected to be easily synthesized from other sequences and error resulted. However, the system indicates locations where the network is uncertain about the regressed output. Qualitative results indicate that errors within the tumour enhancement have associated relatively high uncertainties. This suggests that these uncertainties can be communicated to a clinician or radiologist to indicate trustworthy regions of the synthesized images, and that automatic downstream methods using the synthesized volumes can focus computations on the areas of high confidence, which should be explored in future work.

Table 2. Comparison of multi-class brain tumour segmentation based on S-Net on the BraTS 2017 Validation dataset. The results using all 4 real MRI volumes are compared against replacing 1 real MRI volume with a synthesized MRI volume produced by RS-Net. Notation: Real MR volume (✓), and synthesized MR volume using RS-Net (⊙). Quantitative segmentation results based on Dice coefficients for: enhancing tumor (DE), whole tumor (DT), and tumor core (DC).

	T1	T2	FLAIR	T1ce	DE	DT	DC
Real	✓	✓	✓	✓	**68.2**	**87.9**	**75.7**
T1 synthesis	⊙	✓	✓	✓	67.6	87.9	75.5
T2 synthesis	✓	⊙	✓	✓	66.3	87.3	75.6
FLAIR synthesis	✓	✓	⊙	✓	66.8	83.6	73.1
T1ce synthesis	✓	✓	✓	⊙	24.8	87.3	54.0

Replacing Real with Synthetic MRI Volumes: In Table 2, we compare the tumour segmentation using S-Net in two different testing scenarios, (i) all 4 real MR volumes are provided as input and (ii) 1 real MR volume is replaced with synthesized MR volume for each sequence generated by RS-Net, in turn. We train 4 different RS-Nets to synthesize 4 MR image sequences, where 3 real sequences are presented as input to RS-Net to synthesize the fourth. The synthesized MR volume, along with the 3 real corresponding MR volumes, were then presented to the S-Net previously trained on all four real MRIs. This will allow us to measure quality of the synthesized volume in comparison to the real volume. The resulting labels for BraTS 2017 validation set were uploaded to the BraTS Challenge server, where quantitative segmentation results were provided based on the Dice coefficients for: whole tumor, enhancing tumor, and tumor core. These results (Table 2) indicate that by swapping out real MR volumes with the synthesized T1 or T2 MR volumes generated by the RS-Net leads to comparable brain tumour segmentation performance based on all three reported Dice metrics. For the slightly harder problem of FLAIR synthesis, results indicate a small degradation in tumour segmentation performance for all three Dice metrics. T1ce synthesis results in no loss of whole tumour segmentation performance, but, as predicted, led to a significant reduction in performance in terms of enhancement and necrotic core. This was expected as T1ce is a challenging MRI to synthesize due to its reliance on a contrast agent, which is not used by any other MR sequences.

Effectiveness of Combined Regression-Segmentation Task: RS-Net has two output streams for synthesis and segmentation tasks. To check how RS-Net performs in comparison to a network which is trained only for the task of synthesis, we train a new network (**R-Net**) which is similar to RS-Net but modified such that the segmentation block is removed as well as the additional input to the regression block, and training is based only on weighted MSE. R-Net was trained for the synthesis of all 4 MR image sequences separately, in a leave-

Table 3. Comparison of multi-class brain tumour segmentation results based on S-Net on the BraTS 2017 Validation dataset, where each real MR input volume is replaced by its corresponding synthesized MR volume generated by either RS-Net or R-Net in a leave-one-out fashion. Notation: Real MR volume ($\checkmark$), synthesized MR volume using RS-Net ($\odot$), and R-Net ($\bullet$). Quantitative segmentation results based on Dice coefficients for: enhancing tumor (DE), whole tumor (DT), and tumor core (DC).

	T1	T2	FLAIR	T1ce	DE	DT	DC
Real	$\checkmark$	$\checkmark$	$\checkmark$	$\checkmark$	**68.2**	**87.9**	**75.7**
T1 synthesis	$\odot$	$\checkmark$	$\checkmark$	$\checkmark$	67.6	87.9	75.5
	$\bullet$	$\checkmark$	$\checkmark$	$\checkmark$	67.5	87.8	75.3
T2 synthesis	$\checkmark$	$\odot$	$\checkmark$	$\checkmark$	66.3	87.3	75.6
	$\checkmark$	$\bullet$	$\checkmark$	$\checkmark$	66.1	87.2	75.4
FLAIR synthesis	$\checkmark$	$\checkmark$	$\odot$	$\checkmark$	66.8	83.6	73.1
	$\checkmark$	$\checkmark$	$\bullet$	$\checkmark$	62.9	81.3	71.5
T1ce synthesis	$\checkmark$	$\checkmark$	$\checkmark$	$\odot$	24.8	87.3	54.0
	$\checkmark$	$\checkmark$	$\checkmark$	$\bullet$	24.1	85.9	53.9

one-out approach, and tested for tumor segmentation using S-Net on the BraTS validation dataset exactly as described above. From Table 3, we can observe that R-Net performs comparably to RS-Net, when T1 and T2 are synthesized but shows a small degradation in performance for FLAIR and T1ce synthesis on all three Dice metrics. This shows that performing synthesis and segmentation together allows the network to focus more on tumour part, and in turn gives better quality of the synthesized volume, especially for FLAIR and T1ce.

Table 4. Comparison of multi-class brain tumour segmentation results based on S-Net against the results generated directly from the segmentation module of RS-Net for the BraTS 2017 Validation dataset. Notation: Real MR volume ($\checkmark$), synthesized MR volume using RS-Net ($\odot$), and segmentation output of RS-Net without MR volume ($\times$). Quantitative segmentation results based on Dice coefficients: enhancing tumor (DE), whole tumor (DT), and tumor core (DC).

	T1	T2	FLAIR	T1ce	DE	DT	DC
Real	$\checkmark$	$\checkmark$	$\checkmark$	$\checkmark$	**68.2**	**87.9**	**75.7**
T1 synthesis	$\odot$	$\checkmark$	$\checkmark$	$\checkmark$	67.6	87.9	75.5
	$\times$	$\checkmark$	$\checkmark$	$\checkmark$	66.4	85.2	71.0
T2 synthesis	$\checkmark$	$\odot$	$\checkmark$	$\checkmark$	66.3	87.3	75.6
	$\checkmark$	$\times$	$\checkmark$	$\checkmark$	66.5	87.0	71.1
FLAIR synthesis	$\checkmark$	$\checkmark$	$\odot$	$\checkmark$	66.8	83.6	73.1
	$\checkmark$	$\checkmark$	$\times$	$\checkmark$	70.5	82.6	74.0
T1ce synthesis	$\checkmark$	$\checkmark$	$\checkmark$	$\odot$	24.8	87.3	54.0
	$\checkmark$	$\checkmark$	$\checkmark$	$\times$	23.1	86.5	52.0

Performance of Segmentation Part of RS-Net: One of the advantages of the RS-Net is that, in addition to MRI synthesis, it also provides tumour segmentation labels. In this section, we will analyze this segmentation part of RS-Net (Fig. 1(2)). Table 4 indicates that the segmentation performance based on RS-Net directly is lower than the results based on using all 4 real MR volumes in S-Net, but is generally lower in comparison to the segmentation results when synthesized MR volumes generated by RS-Net is used in place of a real MR volumes. This trend is consistent across all MR image sequences for all three Dice metrics, except for FLAIR where the enhancing and core tumour Dice is higher for segmentation directly from the RS-Net over the segmentation results from S-Net with a synthesized input (for unknown reasons).

4   Conclusions

In this paper, a full resolution 3D end-to-end CNN was developed for the task of MR volume synthesis in the presence of brain tumours. The network was trained for the concurrent tasks of synthesizing a missing MRI sequence and tumour sub-tissue segmentation. Experimental results on BraTS 2015 challenge dataset indicated that the proposed method outperforms all previous methods in terms of traditional evaluation metrics like PSNR and SSIM. The quality of the synthesized images was further evaluated by assessing their effects on the performance in independent tumour segmentation experiments. Experiments on the BraTS 2017 challenge dataset indicated that multi-task learning helps in synthesizing high quality volumes over synthesis alone particularly in more challenging contexts (i.e. FLAIR and T1ce). Results indicated that real MRIs can be replaced with synthesized T1, T2, and FLAIR volumes with minimum degradation in segmentation accuracy, whereas synthesizing T1ce is still too challenging for the task of tumour enhancement segmentation. However, uncertainty measure based on Monte Carlo dropout was shown to be helpful in communicating the confidence in the synthesis results, which will be essential for their adoption by clinicians and downstream automatic methods. The code for the proposed method is available here: https://github.com/RagMeh11/RS-Net.

Acknowledgment. This work was supported by a Canadian Natural Science and Engineering Research Council (NSERC) Collaborative Research and Development Grant (CRDPJ 505357 - 16) and Synaptive Medical. We gratefully acknowledge the support of NVIDIA Corporation for the donation of the Titan X Pascal GPU used for this research.

References

1. Menze, B.H., et al.: The multimodal brain tumor image segmentation benchmark (BRATS). IEEE TMI **34**, 1993 (2015)
2. Havaei, M., Guizard, N., Chapados, N., Bengio, Y.: HeMIS: hetero-modal image segmentation. In: Ourselin, S., Joskowicz, L., Sabuncu, M.R., Unal, G., Wells, W. (eds.) MICCAI 2016. LNCS, vol. 9901, pp. 469–477. Springer, Cham (2016). https://doi.org/10.1007/978-3-319-46723-8_54

3. van Tulder, G., de Bruijne, M.: Why does synthesized data improve multi-sequence classification? In: Navab, N., Hornegger, J., Wells, W.M., Frangi, A.F. (eds.) MICCAI 2015. LNCS, vol. 9349, pp. 531–538. Springer, Cham (2015). https://doi.org/10.1007/978-3-319-24553-9_65

4. Jog, A., et al.: Random forest regression for magnetic resonance image synthesis. Med. Image Anal. **35**, 475–488 (2017)

5. Roy, S., Carass, A., Prince, J.: A compressed sensing approach for MR tissue contrast synthesis. In: Székely, G., Hahn, H.K. (eds.) IPMI 2011. LNCS, vol. 6801, pp. 371–383. Springer, Heidelberg (2011). https://doi.org/10.1007/978-3-642-22092-0_31

6. Van Nguyen, H., Zhou, K., Vemulapalli, R.: Cross-domain synthesis of medical images using efficient location-sensitive deep network. In: Navab, N., Hornegger, J., Wells, W.M., Frangi, A.F. (eds.) MICCAI 2015. LNCS, vol. 9349, pp. 677–684. Springer, Cham (2015). https://doi.org/10.1007/978-3-319-24553-9_83

7. Zhang, R., Isola, P., Efros, A.A.: Colorful image colorization. In: Leibe, B., Matas, J., Sebe, N., Welling, M. (eds.) ECCV 2016. LNCS, vol. 9907, pp. 649–666. Springer, Cham (2016). https://doi.org/10.1007/978-3-319-46487-9_40

8. Isola, P., et al.: Image-to-image translation with conditional adversarial networks. arXiv preprint, 1 July 2017

9. Chartsias, A., et al.: Multimodal MR synthesis via modality-invariant latent representation. IEEE TMI **37**, 803–814 (2017)

10. Wolterink, J.M., Dinkla, A.M., Savenije, M.H.F., Seevinck, P.R., van den Berg, C.A.T., Išgum, I.: Deep MR to CT synthesis using unpaired data. In: Tsaftaris, S.A., Gooya, A., Frangi, A.F., Prince, J.L. (eds.) SASHIMI 2017. LNCS, vol. 10557, pp. 14–23. Springer, Cham (2017). https://doi.org/10.1007/978-3-319-68127-6_2

11. Gal, Y., Ghahramani, Z.: Dropout as a Bayesian approximation: representing model uncertainty in deep learning. In: ICML, pp. 1050–1059 (2016)

12. Çiçek, Ö., Abdulkadir, A., Lienkamp, S.S., Brox, T., Ronneberger, O.: 3D U-Net: learning dense volumetric segmentation from sparse annotation. In: Ourselin, S., Joskowicz, L., Sabuncu, M.R., Unal, G., Wells, W. (eds.) MICCAI 2016. LNCS, vol. 9901, pp. 424–432. Springer, Cham (2016). https://doi.org/10.1007/978-3-319-46723-8_49

13. Ulyanov, D., et al.: Instance normalization: the missing ingredient for fast stylization. arXiv preprint arXiv:1607.08022

14. Srivastava, N., et al.: Dropout: a simple way to prevent neural networks from overfitting. JMLR **15**(1), 1929–1958 (2014)

15. Kingma, D.P., Ba, J.: Adam: a method for stochastic optimization. arXiv preprint arXiv:1412.6980

16. Wang, Z., et al.: Image quality assessment: from error visibility to structural similarity. TIP **13**(4), 600–612 (2004)

Generating Magnetic Resonance Spectroscopy Imaging Data of Brain Tumours from Linear, Non-linear and Deep Learning Models

Nathan Olliverre[1]([✉]), Guang Yang[3,4], Gregory Slabaugh[1],
Constantino Carlos Reyes-Aldasoro[2], and Eduardo Alonso[1]

[1] Department of Computer Science, City University of London,
London EC1V 0HB, UK
nathan.olliverre@city.ac.uk
[2] Department of Electrical Engineering, City University of London,
London EC1V 0HB, UK
[3] Cardiovascular Biomedical Research Unit, Royal Brompton Hospital,
London SW3 6NP, UK
[4] National Heart and Lung Institute, Imperial College London,
London SW7 2AZ, UK

Abstract. Magnetic Resonance Spectroscopy (MRS) provides valuable information to help with the identification and understanding of brain tumors, yet MRS is not a widely available medical imaging modality. Aiming to counter this issue, this research draws on the advancements in machine learning techniques in other fields for the generation of artificial data. The generated methods were tested through the evaluation of their output against that of a real-world labelled MRS brain tumor data-set. Furthermore the resultant output from the generative techniques were each used to train separate traditional classifiers which were tested on a subset of the real MRS brain tumor dataset. The results suggest that there exist methods capable of producing accurate, ground truth based MRS voxels. These findings indicate that through generative techniques, large datasets can be made available for training deep, learning models for the use in brain tumor diagnosis.

1 Introduction

Within the UK over 11,000 brain tumor cases are diagnosed each year [5]. The survival rate and period of progression have been shown to improve with treatment [22]. The process to determine treatment can be difficult and time consuming [21], this is further complicated due to limited numbers of staff available to perform these tasks [9]. These tasks also lead to the most errors in diagnosis [9]. The automation of the tasks involved in diagnosis could help to increase the accuracy and reduce the time it takes for the application of treatment to a patient.

© Springer Nature Switzerland AG 2018
A. Gooya et al. (Eds.): SASHIMI 2018, LNCS 11037, pp. 130–138, 2018.
https://doi.org/10.1007/978-3-030-00536-8_14

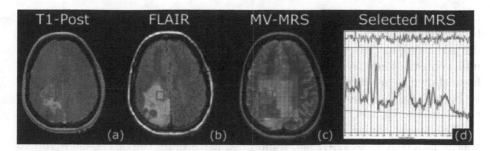

Fig. 1. Example of a T1-Post MRI (a), Fluid-Attenuated Inversion Recovery (FLAIR) MRI (b), Multi-Voxel MRS Heatmap overlaid on FLAIR (c) and the selected Single-Voxel MRS highlighted in each of the images as the red square (d) (Color figure online).

Magnetic Resonance Spectroscopy (MRS), also known as MR Spectroscopic Imaging (MRSI) or Chemical Shift Imaging (CSI), provides a non-invasive method for the diagnosis of human tissue such as lung, bone or brain matter. Similar to MR Imaging (MRI), MRS is based upon the principles of Nuclear Magnetic Resonance (NMR) [2]; however, whereas MRI uses the resultant proton signals to create detailed graphical output, MRS uses the signals to determine the quantity in parts per million (ppm) of various metabolites within cells [10] which can be seen in the example shown in Fig. 1. One area in which MRS has been shown to provide valuable insights is in the case of brain tumors [11]. In medical imaging research, MRS has proven to produce accurate results in identification of tumor grade classification [11,20].

Current state-of-the-art computer vision models in medical imaging have begun to utilize the advancements made in machine learning, specifically in the field of deep learning [14]. These deep learning models take advantage of multi-layered networks to extract feature information from the input data. To power the ability for these deep models to extract such feature-rich information, large swaths of data are required [13]. This can be an obstacle in the medical imaging field as restrictions in data protection [7] along with non-standardized practices makes it difficult to collect the required amount of data to work with deep learning models. To be able to apply current state-of-the-art classifiers to MRS brain tumor images more data is required, hence techniques to fabricate or generate data are essential.

Advancements in computer vision and machine learning have also given the rise to accurate generative techniques for the creation of artificial data. One such generative technique is Generative Adversarial Networks (GANs) [8] which have been developed to help create more domain specific/accurate artificial data. GANs use multiple models working against each other to create accurate data, with one model (Generator) attempting to produce artificial data capable of "fooling" a model trained to determine "real" from "fake" data (Discriminator). By using approaches such as GANs the process of creating data that adheres to the domain can be achieved. Recently, variations of the original

GAN model have been developed to produce better results. The Deeply Convolutional GAN (DCGAN) [17], which takes into account the improvements that deep learning models have shown against their traditional counterparts uses a multi-convolutional layered Generator and Discriminator. Although GANs have been shown to produce accurate results in various fields [17,19] they are known to be unstable and hard to train [3] whereas their more linear counterparts are considered to be easier to train but less expressive.

This paper applies three of the state-of-the-art methods in generating synthetic data (GAN, DCGAN and a modified MRS brain tumor classifier [16]) to the domain of MRS for review. To determine the accuracy of the artificial data created each generated dataset was used to train a Random Forest for the classification of brain tumors. The results from the trained Random Forest classifiers were bench-marked against the results of one trained on the real MRS images.

2   Materials and Methods

2.1   Materials

The MRS dataset used in this study was obtained by St. George's University London and consisted of a single-voxel MRS training and testing set. Both the test and training sets were acquired using a GE Signa Horizon 1.5T MR system with a Repetition Time (TR) and a short Echo Time (TE) of 2000 ms and 30 ms respectively. A Point-Resolved spectroscopic sequence protocol was used to acquire the training and test dataset. The World Health Organization classifies tumours into 4 grades (WHO) [6]: Grades I - IV, with GI and GII being deemed low grade tumors and GIII and GIV said to be high grade, malignant tumors. The composition of the training and test dataset was 137 samples. Of the training set 70 were classified as healthy tissue, 20 as GII (low grade), 10 as GIII and 20 GIV (high grade). The test set consisted of 9 healthy, 3 low grade and 5 high grade which were taken through random sampling of the entire dataset prior to training. Due to the similarity between GIII and GIV tumour tissue in MRS imaging, the GIII data was merged with the GIV data by labelling each as high grade. Figure 2 illustrates MRS spectra of different grades.

The positioning for every scan captured in the dataset was placed on a homogeneous, representative tumor region determined by an expert using post-Gd contrast T1w, T2w and FLAIR structural contrast images alongside the relevant histopathological information. This was to ensure accuracy within the training data and that there was a heterogeneity of MRS characteristics represented within each voxel scanned. The individual labels for the data were achieved via the diagnosis of a biopsy by a practiced physician in which the clinical, radiological and histopathological information of each patient was incorporated to the diagnosis.

The nature of MRS data is high-dimensional (of roughly 1,024 dimensions) thus a reduction with Principal Component Analysis (PCA) was applied to explore the data, see Fig. 3. Clustering with k-means results in a good separation of the classes, especially between healthy and high grade tissue (Fig. 3b).

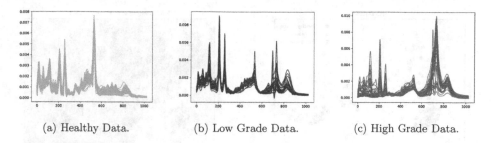

(a) Healthy Data.   (b) Low Grade Data.   (c) High Grade Data.

Fig. 2. Illustration of the MRS spectra grouped into a healthy (green), (b) low grade (blue) and (c) high grade (red) tumor tissue. Peaks correspond to metabolites in the region of interest. (Color figure online)

2.2 Methods

This study took a three step approach. First, three different models (GAN, DCGAN and a generative adaptation of PMM) were used to generated synthetic MRS images based off of the training -MRS- dataset. Second, these samples were then each used to train a Random Forest to be able to classify MRS images as either healthy, low or high grade tissue. Finally, the results from the Random Forest classifiers were then analyzed and the synthetic data from the generative models were compared against the mean signal of the training dataset classes.

The GAN model used in this study, based on [8], had a generator comprised of a fully connected input layer which accepted a random value vector of size 100, with a hidden layer of 1,024 nodes in size using rectified exponential linear (ReLU) [15] as the activation function with the output layer having 1,024 nodes but utilizing TanH [1] as the activation function. The discriminator consisted of a linear input layer which took in an MRS image of 1,024 values, followed by a hidden layer consisting of 1,024 nodes using LeakyReLU [1] as the activation function, the output layer was a singular sigmoidal node [18] activation. The full model was trained on each class of tissue for over 150,000 epochs using the Adam optimizer [12].

Compared to GANs, DCGANs use a deeper learning architecture which normally requires more data. To try and generate more expressive and domain accurate data, alterations were required to the training of the network to accommodate the limited data. The training process was modified to not take random batch samples but to deliberately take the full set of the data available for training at each epoch. The samples were then normalized with batch normalization. The architecture for the generator used in the study was a fully connected input layer comprised of 2048 nodes followed by four transposed one-dimensional convolutional layers using LeakyReLU as the activation function for all but the output layer which used TanH. The discriminator was the inverse with the first four layers being one-dimensional convolutions (using LeakyReLU as the activation function) followed by a single Sigmodial output node. Similar to the GAN model the DCGAN model was trained for at least 250,000 epochs on each tissue class.

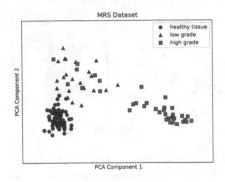
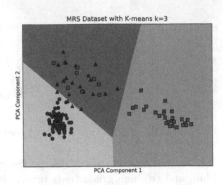

(a) PCA applied with two components.   (b) K-means clustering applied.

Fig. 3. Application of PCA to the MRS dataset with the first two components used (a) followed by k-means clustering (b).

GANs are a non-linear method for the generation of data which, theoretically, should lead to more expressive data over that of more linear methods but to do so requires larger amounts of training data. To test the benefits, a comparison to a linear based generator in the study was required. For medical imaging data, factors such as patient orientation and relationship between values matters. Therefore, testing requires a method which can generate data that adheres to the domain. The selected method for this study was the Pairwise Mixture Model.

The Pairwise Mixture Model (PMM) [16] is a model for representing different brain tissue from MRS images and based on the work by Asad et al. [4], the purpose of which was to solve the problem of the heterogeneity of tissue types found within multi-voxel MRS images. The possible types were defined as normal, low (GI and GII type brain tumour tissue) and high (GIII and GIV brain tumour tissue). Each tissue model is expressed as a mean signal and the variation around the mean, calculated from applying PCA to a labelled dataset of homogeneous MRS images each relating to a specific grade. The models could then be as defined:

$$m_i(t) = \mu_i(t) + \sum \alpha_i e_{ik}(t), \qquad (1)$$

where μ_i is the mean signal, α_i and e_i respectively are the alpha weight coefficients and eigenvectors - which encode the variation around the mean signal - with K representing the number of eigenvectors determined for model m_i. To calculate the amount of each tissue type found within a certain voxel the assumption that each voxel was a weighted sum of the possible tissue types gives the following:

$$s(t) = w_n m_n(t) + w_l m_l(t) + w_h m_h(t), \qquad (2)$$

which can then be viewed as an optimization problem where:

$$E = \int [x(t) - s(t)]^2 dt + \int [\sum_j s(t) - s_j(t)]^2 dt, \quad (3)$$

with j representing the available surrounding model signals of $s(t)$.

The estimated coefficients can be considered to represent the amount of each tissue type (normal, low or high) found within a voxel.

By taking the models of the various tissue types from the PMM, it is straightforward to see how by varying the value of the coefficients of the models it is possible to create data that holds to the original domain. There is a limit to the amount of possibly created data (c^3 where c represents the coefficients) but it is still enough to train a classifier model with a deep learning architecture, based on the generated data alone.

The testing of the generated data from each network used a set of simple, shallow Random Forest classifiers which were constructed and trained on the generated data from the GAN, DCGAN and the PMM generation method. A Random Forest was also trained on the training dataset alone as a control set. The Random Forest classifiers were then tested on the MRS image test set with the classification accuracy results recorded and examined. Furthermore the generated MRS images were compared to the mean signal from the training dataset for comparison to determine the adherence to the domain and possibility of expressiveness.

3 Results

Each model, the GAN, DCGAN and PMM generator, was trained on the MRS single-voxel training dataset for each class (normal, low and high). The GAN and DCGAN each had the architecture detailed in Sect. 2.2.

Table 1. Table showing the resultant classification accuracy from the set of Random Forests trained on the generated data from the GAN, PMM and the DCGAN compared to that of a Random Forest trained on only the real, labelled training dataset (GT).

Grade	PMM	GAN	DCGAN	GT
Healthy	93%	97.5%	71%	96%
Low	96%	97%	66%	95%
High	93%	93%	71%	95%

From the results shown in Table 1 the GAN produced higher accuracy in the Random Forest classifier trained on its data than with the DCGAN generated method for low grade tumor patients and for normal (healthy) tissue. The classifier trained on PMM data produced higher accuracy for low grade tumor

Table 2. Table showing the mean squared error of the linear differences between the generated signals and the mean signal of the ground truth data for each class

Grade	PMM	GAN	DCGAN
Healthy	0.002	1.021	5.148
Low	0.004	2.044	4.063
High	0.071	3.029	12.001

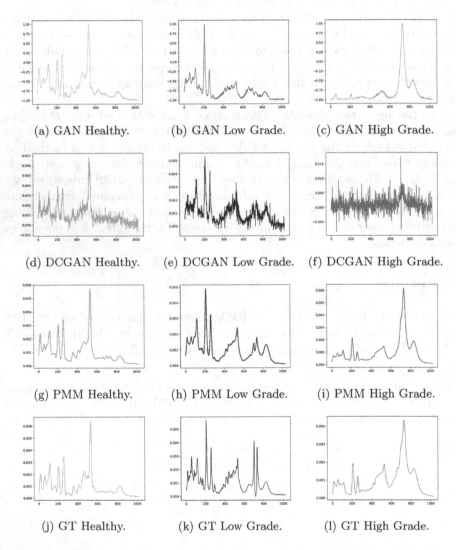

(a) GAN Healthy.   (b) GAN Low Grade.   (c) GAN High Grade.

(d) DCGAN Healthy.   (e) DCGAN Low Grade.   (f) DCGAN High Grade.

(g) PMM Healthy.   (h) PMM Low Grade.   (i) PMM High Grade.

(j) GT Healthy.   (k) GT Low Grade.   (l) GT High Grade.

Fig. 4. Artificially generated MRS signals of healthy (green), low grade (blue) and high grade (red) tumor tissue produced from the PMM generation method (g, h, i), the GAN (a, b, c) and the DCGAN (d, e, f) compared with samples from the ground truth dataset (j, k, l). (Color figure online)

patients over that of the ground truth. The DCGAN produced the worst results over all tissue types.

The most variation within the resultant signals can be seen from both GAN methods, however, the GAN appears to cohere closer to the shape of the real MRS signals as shown in Fig. 4, this can be shown through the deltas between signals shown in Table 2.

4 Conclusions

This paper examines the possibility of generating MRS brain tumor images from limited and uneven data through one state-of-the-art generation technique, a deeper version of the same model and a modified MRS brain tumor model (GAN, DCGAN and PMM respectively). The results showed that the generated data could train a shallow Random Forest classifier to accurately determine the grades of brain tissue to the same level of one trained on real MRS data. The GAN trained model produced higher accuracy in testing and shows the expressiveness and capability in adversarial networks whereas the DCGAN model produced the lowest accuracy in classification as well as in similarity to the training data, highlighting the need for larger amounts of data when working with deep learning models. The linear model was able to produce spectra that were closer in appearance to the mean signal of the training dataset. The next stage is to examine the generated voxels by a domain expert to acknowledge their potential accuracy and expressiveness, the analysis drawn can then be used to determine what needs to be done in order to have the generated data successfully train a deep learning model for the classification of MRS images.

Acknowledgements. We would like to thank Professor Franklyn Howe at St George's, University of London, for the brain tumour MR data used in this research as well as his insights into MRS. We are also grateful for the hardware provided to us by NVIDIA that was used in this research.

References

1. Agostinelli, F., et al.: Learning activation functions to improve deep neural networks. In: arXiv:1412.6830 [cs, stat], 21 December 21 2014
2. Andrew, E.R.: Nuclear magnetic resonance and the brain. Brain Topograph. 5(2), 129–133 (1992)
3. Arjovsky, M., et al.: Towards principled methods for training generative adversarial networks. In: arXiv:1701.04862 [cs, stat], 17 January 2017
4. Asad, M., et al.: Supervised partial volume effect unmixing for brain tumor characterization using multi-voxel MR spectroscopic imaging. In: 2016 IEEE 13th International Symposium on Biomedical Imaging (ISBI). 2016 IEEE 13th International Symposium on Biomedical Imaging (ISBI), pp. 436–439, April 2016
5. CRUK Cancer Research UK: Brain, other CNS and intracranial tumours statistics. Cancer Research UK, 14 May 2015. http://www.cancerresearchuk.org/health-professional/cancer-statistics/statistics-by-cancer-type/brain-other-cns-and-intra cranial-tumours. Accessed 03 Jan 2018

6. Centre international de recherche sur le cancer et al. (eds.): Pathology and genetics of tumours of the lung, pleura, thymus and heart. IARC Press, Lyon (2004). OCLC: 492146534

7. Cios, K.J., et al.: Uniqueness of medical data mining. Artif. Intell. Med. **26**(1), 1–24 (2002). Medical Data Mining and Knowledge Discovery

8. Goodfellow, I., et al.: Generative adversarial nets. In: Ghahramani, Z., et al. (eds.) Advances in Neural Information Processing Systems 27, pp. 2672–2680. Curran Associates Inc. (2014)

9. Grant, R.: Overview: brain tumour diagnosis and management/Royal College of Physicians guidelines. J. Neurol. Neurosurg. Psychiat. **75**(Suppl. 2), ii18–ii23 (2004)

10. Gujar, S.K., et al.: Magnetic resonance spectroscopy. J. Neuro-Ophthalmol. **25**(3), 217 (2015)

11. Howe, F.A., et al.: 1H MR spectroscopy of brain tumours and masses. NMR Biomed. **16**(3), 123–131 (2003)

12. Kingma, D.P., et al.: Adam: a method for stochastic optimization. In: arXiv:1412.6980, 22 December 2014

13. LeCun, Y.: Deep learning. Nature **521**(7553), 436–444 (2015)

14. Litjens, G., et al.: A survey on deep learning in medical image analysis. Med. Image Anal. **42**, 60–88 (2017)

15. Nair, V., et al.: Rectified linear units improve restricted Boltzmann machines. In: Proceedings of the 27th International Conference on International Conference on Machine Learning, ICML 2010, pp. 807–814. Omnipress, Madison (2010)

16. Olliverre, N., et al.: Pairwise mixture model for unmixing partial volume effect in multi-voxel MR spectroscopy of brain tumour patients. In: Medical Imaging 2017: Computer-Aided Diagnosis, 3 March 2017, vol. 10134. International Society for Optics and Photonics (2017). 101341R

17. Radford, A., et al.: Unsupervised representation learning with deep convolutional generative adversarial networks. In: arXiv:1511.06434 [cs], 19 November 2015

18. Rumelhart, D.E.: Learning representations by back-propagating errors. Nature **323**(6088), 533–536 (1986)

19. Salimans, T., et al.: Improved techniques for training GANs. In: arXiv:1606.03498 [cs], 10 June 2016

20. Sibtain, N.A.: The clinical value of proton magnetic resonance spectroscopy in adult brain tumours. Clin. Radiol. **62**(2), 109–119 (2007)

21. Yang, G.: Discrete wavelet transform-based whole-spectral and subspectral analysis for improved brain tumor clustering using single Voxel MR spectroscopy. IEEE Trans. Biomed. Eng. **62**(12), 2860–2866 (2015)

22. Zacharaki, E.I.: Classification of brain tumor type and grade using MRI texture and shape in a machine learning scheme. Magn. Reson. Med. **62**(6), 1609–1618 (2009)

Author Index

Printed in the United States
By Bookmasters